Dementia care and the general practitioner

Other books by the same author:

Dementia: Management for nurses and community care workers
Travel and Health in the Elderly
Health Hazard and the Higher Risk Traveller
Pitstops and Pitfalls: A Health Guide for Older Travellers

Dementia care and the general practitioner

by

Dr Iain B McIntosh

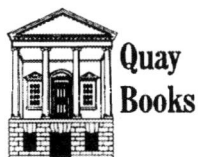

Quay Books, Mark Allen Publishing Group Limited
Jesses Farm, Snow Hill, Dinton
Salisbury, Wiltshire SP3 5HN

British Library Cataloguing-in-Publication Data

A catalogue record is available for this book

© Mark Allen Publishing Ltd, 1998
ISBN 1 85642 048 5

All rights reserved. No part of this publication may be reproduced, stored in a retrieval system, or transmitted in any form or by any means, electronic, mechanical, photocopying, recording or otherwise, without prior permission from the publishers.

Printed in the UK by Antony Rowe Limited, Chippenham, Wiltshire

Contents

	Acknowledgements	vii
1	The daunting demands of dementia care — a therapeutic challenge	1
2	**Dementia — the syndrome**	6
	Definition	6
	The size of the problem	7
	Pathology	9
	Causes of dementia	14
	Non-ATD dementias	17
3	**The disease process**	21
	A progressive disease	21
	Clinical presentation	22
	Emotional changes	24
	Cognitive changes	24
	Behavioural changes	24
4	**Making the diagnosis**	28
	Detection and early diagnosis	28
	Advantages to patient, carer and doctor	30
	Assessment procedures	36
	Onward referral of the patient	45
	Memory clinics	47
5	**The differential diagnosis**	49
	DSM-IV criteria for diagnosis of Alzheimer's disease	52
	Confusional states	55
	Depression and dementia	57
	Memory tests	63
6	**The GP's role in management**	69
	Guidelines for good practice	72
	The primary health care team's role in management	75

	Nursing home care	78
7	**Roles of the care team**	82
8	**Drug management of dementias and behaviour problems**	94
	Drug research approaches to ATD	95
	Acetylcholine esterase inhibitors	98
	Drug treatment for depression	100
	Antipschotic or neuroleptic drug use in dementia	102
	Drug therapy for sleep disturbance	106
9	**Non-drug interventions in dementia management**	110
	Reality orientation	116
	Reminiscence therapy	117
	Validation therapy	118
	Cognitive deficiency and behavioural problems	119
10	**Management of challenging behaviour**	123
	Anger and hostility	124
	Wandering	125
	Urinary and faecal incontinence	130
11	**Caring for the carer**	136
	Depression in carers	139
	Patient abuse	148
	Financial and legal concerns	152

Conclusion 159
Appendixes
   1. Mini-Mental State Examination 160
   2. Hachinski Ischaemic Score 163
   3. Activites of daily living: Barthel Index 164
   4. Over-75s assessment profile 165
   5. Abbreviated Mental Test 170
   6. Geriatric depression scale 171
References 173
Index 184

Acknowledgements

The author would like to thank Professor Mary Marshall and the staff of the Dementia Services Development Centre, University of Stirling, for their support while writing this book.

1
The daunting demands of dementia care — a therapeutic challenge

One paper on dementia is published every five hours (Kist and Hastie, 1995). Despite intense research effort, this mental disorder largely remains an enigma, of obscure aetiology, difficult to diagnose and with limited drug treatment potential. Its optimal therapeutic management can be a challenge for GPs and the primary care team.

People with dementia have a progressive disease which ultimately leads to premature death. They and their family carers may present many physical, psychological, emotional and behavioural problems, in surgery consultations and home visits, when residing in the community. Many patients occupy nursing homes or longstay units where they frequently remain the responsibility of the local GP.

A substantial part of the general population consists of older people. There is an exponential increase in the prevalence of dementia with increasing age. With the population of elderly people, especially the very old, set to increase over the next decade, there are likely to be many patients with dementia seeking professional care. The provisions of the NHS and Community Care Act,1990, implemented in 1993, make it likely that they shall be encouraged to live in their own homes. They and their carers remain the responsibility of the family doctor and the community care team.

Family doctors are key personnel in the provision of health care for patients and carers coping with the consequences of dementia. Eighty per cent of people with this illness live at home, many on their own. The Secretaries of State for Health and Social Security inquiry of 1989 identified the GP as having a vital role in community care for people with severe mental illness and recognised that only a minority of GPs have any formal training in psychiatry.

A diagnosis of dementia often triggers feelings of hopelessness and helplessness in doctors and nurses. GPs and carers have low expectations of what primary medical care has to offer people with dementia and family doctors perform poorly in identifying those with early and established dementia (Ledesert *et al*, 1994). Figures from recent studies (O'Connor *et al*, 1988) found that GPs in England were able to identify only 58% of cases but misdiagnosis of dementia was also not uncommon (Cooper, 1992).

People with dementia are often old, communicate poorly and even when identified can easily receive low priority in GP support and management (McIntosh et al, 1997).

All too frequently the family carers' problems go unrecognised and unsupported. Good management in dementia care can be a drain on economic resources, and the advent of 'fundholding' to general medical practice threatens the provision of services that these patients require and deserve. People with dementia are known to be disproportionately heavy users of the health services. However, they do not always receive the quality of care that their condition merits.

Many of their problems result from loss of mental function, but others are caused by the family's reaction and professional carers' response to the illness. These interrelationship difficulties, if appreciated and understood by the professional carer, may be ameliorated or resolved resulting in an improved quality of life for both patient and carer. GPs have an important and crucial role in making an early diagnosis of dementia by considering and excluding differential diagnoses, arranging and coordinating appropriate support for the patient and family carer, and providing continuity of care in this progressive, terminal illness which can devastate the patient and endanger the health of the carer.

Many studies have shown a shortfall in the quality of care given to dementia patients by GPs and the primary health care team. There is a failure to identify the disease, an absence of multidisciplinary assessment, a lack of co-ordinated care and little attention given to the needs of carers. Clinicians appear to have an aversion to early intervention, possibly because of the fear that early detection of dementia merely increases the demand on overburdened services.

Misdiagnoses are not uncommon and the condition is often diagnosed when dementia is not present and other functional disorders are present or coexist. Lack of time, poor expertise, difficulties in making the diagnosis, no perceived advantage in early diagnosis, inadequate provision of support services have all been cited as reasons for the variable response in care. The GP is, nevertheless, of vital importance as key worker, gatekeeper and organiser in the good management of patients with a dementing process.

The hospice movement has brought a radical change in attitude to management in terminal cancer care. The quality of cancer sufferers' lives has been much improved and professional advice and support have dramatically changed for the better. Dementia is also a terminal condition, unfortunately placed at the opposite end of the medical treatment spectrum, and still suffering from therapeutic nihilism, reactive crisis intervention and the failure of health professionals to adopt a holistic approach to management. Recent innovations in drug therapy are slowing the advance of the disease. One of the many drugs being researched may well bring the breakthrough required to halt the inexorable progression of this condition.

The wind of change is blowing upon the management of dementia. A new culture in the care process has taken root, with the recognition that dementing patients are people with their own individual personhood who, given good supportive care, can retain skills, personalities and a quality of life which should not be denied them.

'A major element in the incapacity of many people with dementia is the way we relate to them, a problem that is ours and not theirs. If we accept dementia to be a disability then we can adopt a rehabilitative approach to management.'

(Marshall, 1994)

The nihilistic approach to dementia, a product of patient institutional incarceration of yesteryear, is sadly all too common today. Carers and health care associations, such as The Alzheimer's Disease Society, are constantly criticising the anachronistic attitudes of doctors to dementia diagnosis and care, and demanding that these be replaced by a more positive outlook regarding management, incorporating:

- early recognition of possible dementia cases
- exclusion of presenting treatable disorders
- identification of need
- creation of a care management plan
- provision of support services.

Adoption of these tenets will ensure that patients and carers receive the consideration they deserve.

Family doctors tend to delay advising patients and carers of a diagnosis of dementia. While this may be due to concern regarding the definitive diagnosis, by so doing they are depriving those involved of early advice and support when it is often badly needed. The lack of a curative or ameliorative drug therapy, the psychiatric, physical and social demands of the disease and difficulties in referral and provision of support services have led to many GPs viewing people with dementia as 'heartsink patients'. Each person with the condition does, however, remain a unique personality, with an individual life history and the ability to enter form relationships.

Each case will differ in terms of mental deterioration, rate of decline, loss of faculties and behaviour responses. Patients will be affected by the illness in different ways. Each individual creates a challenge in terms of active therapeutic management and support provision. A personalised management plan is required which should involve multidisciplinary assessment from different members of the primary care team. GPs cannot escape the demands of dementia but, if committed to early intervention, planned management and active therapy, can bring quality of care and an enlightened approach which will enhance the lives of patients and carers.

Planned intervention will often avert the crisis intervention required of the GP at antisocial hours. With appropriate delegation to the primary care team for support, the time and effort devoted to a committed interventionist approach rather than a demand-led response to dementia care may save many crisis response hours 'on call' when time is at a premium. Early assessment and monitoring of patient and family health and the carer situation can prompt anticipatory guidance, provide information, and trigger social support and appropriate referral. This programme may avert a crisis and unrealistic demands for GP response — unwelcome intrusions when doctors are currently experiencing increasing personal stress. Such an approach can diminish the anxiety— provoking features of caring for people with dementia and, if properly orchestrated, may decrease practice workload (McIntosh et al, 1988)

Lack of training and expertise in this field, difficulties in assessment and the lack of diagnostic confidence have been identified as reasons for GPs' disinterest in the disease (Alzheimer's Disease Society, 1995). This book endeavours to address these issues pragmatically and point the way to enlightened therapeutic management for patients with dementia, whose illness robs them of the ability to ensure that they get the care which their relentlessly progressive condition deserves.

Many people with dementia retain some residual rationality. Although mentally impaired, most still have preferences that merit consideration by professional carers. Those involved should therefore endeavour to find out why people are behaving in a particular fashion. Reasons for the behaviour should be sought so that something can be done to try to change the unacceptable behaviour. The technique of reality orientation first drew attention to the possibility that people with dementia could learn and be helped to adjust to everyday reality.

An increasing focus on newer therapeutic manoeuvres such as validation therapy has shown some may bring improvement in behaviour and wellbeing. There is now an appreciation that people with dementia retain some degree of brain function which may be utilised to the patient's and carer's advantage. Dealing with the immediate medical or physical problem is not the GP's sole responsibility; a global assessment of residual functional capacity, the maximisation of retained skills and consideration of the patient's feelings and personhood are now mandatory in the provision of good dementia care. An enlightened attitude, commitment to optimal care, and a multidisciplinary approach to the provision of support can facilitate a satisfying and satisfactory outcome. These are the prerequisites for overcoming the challenge and daunting demands of dementia.

2
Dementia — the syndrome

Definition

This is a group of diseases associated with progressive, chronic disturbance of intellectual function which results in global deterioration of memory and thinking, sufficient to disturb function in activities of daily living (Gurland, 1983).

Dementia is a syndrome of progressive cerebral failure (Shua-haim, 1996) where consciousness is unimpaired. It involves a decline in cognitive and non-cognitive functions. A diagnosis of dementia should be considered when such symptoms persist for more than six months.

The change in intellectual function can bring disturbance in recall, reasoning, judgment, learning, abstract thought, perception and language. Non-cognitive symptoms involve personality and affect behaviour which lead to an inability to meet the demands of:

- occupation
- social environment
- activities of daily living.

A diagnosis of dementia requires that:

1. The cognitive impairment must be acquired, to distinguish it from mental symptoms demonstrated by a person of developmental subnormal intelligence.
2. The cognitive impairment must be general, to distinguish it from focal defects such as dysphasia.
3. There should be normal alertness to distinguish it from confusional state (Rossor *et al*, 1984).

Presentation can be variable but involves:

- loss of skills
- deterioration in memory
- deterioration in self-care
- unusual behaviour inappropriate to that individual
- altered affect

- personality change
- disturbed thinking
- confusional state.

Changes can be subtle, intermittent, transitory, limited in focus and gradual in appearance. The patient may initially try to cover up deficits to avoid embarrassment. Dating the beginning of the syndrome may be difficult. Brain damage may have been going on for several years without perceptible effect until compensating mechanisms are lost.

Inexorably, however, the process progresses and the syndrome becomes more apparent to carer and observer. Frequently, a behavioural, medical or social crisis brings the condition to the attention of the primary care team. Early recognition of cases, proactive intervention and good care management should pre-empt crisis intervention requests from GPs, which are still a common feature of medical practice.

The size of the problem

Dementia is only one of numerous diseases which present to the GP and may attract scant professional attention. Its demands, however can be disproportionate to the prevalence of the disorder.

In a GP list of 1600-2000 patients there may be about 20 patients with dementia, although GPs with a high proportion of elderly patients and nursing home responsibilities will be responsible for many more. As only 4% of patients with dementia are under 65 years of age (early onset dementia), most patients with dementia are likely to be in the older age groups. With the proportion of elderly in the population set to rise and many people living longer, numbers are likely to increase further by the turn of the century. Since 5-7% of patients on GP lists are over 75 years of age as many as 10% of patients in the older age categories may suffer from this disease. The prevalence rate in Scotland in 1991 was estimated at 9.6 per thousand with 49 000 cases in the Scottish population of 5 million and 550 000 in the population of England (Alzheimer's Disease Society, England, 1993). A 12% increase in new cases is expected by the year 2001 (Jorm and Korten, 1988).

Four out of five people who suffer from dementia live at home and are likely to be the responsibility of the local doctor. Home residence does not necessarily mean mild mental impairment. The provisions of the Community Care Act of 1991 mean that many moderate to severe mentally impaired, dementing patients will remain in the community, where some will inevitably live until they die. The burden on the carer can and does create stress, anxiety and illness, which means that the GP has to deal with the needs and expectations of both patient and carer.

Patients with early-onset dementia in particular have disproportionately higher morbidity than do older dementing patients, and create more social crisis demands which are poorly managed by GPs (Newens *et al*, 1994).

The prevalence of dementia rises exponentially with age and roughly doubles with every five years increase in age (Jorm and Korten, 1988). The total disease duration for a typical patient with Alzheimer's-type dementia (ATD) before death intervenes is 8.5 years (Jost and Grossberg, 1995).

It is anticipated that one in three people over 85 will suffer from dementia. The prevalence of dementia is 2% in those aged 65–69 years, rising to 20% in the 85–89 years age group.

Of the 80% of demented patients living at home, 23% will be living alone, creating individual problems. The situation is not all gloom and doom, however, as even after 90 years of life, two out of three people are likely to be cognitively unimpaired (Ott and Breteler, 1995).

Demographic trends

Old people

Projections of the UK population suggest a shift towards a less youth dominated structure with an expansion in over 75 year olds. The numbers of older people in the population are expected to rise for several years into the 21st century (Figure 2.1).

Dementia

Dementia is not a disease but a consequence of a variety of different diseases, with Alzheimer's disease responsible for a substantial number of the cases.

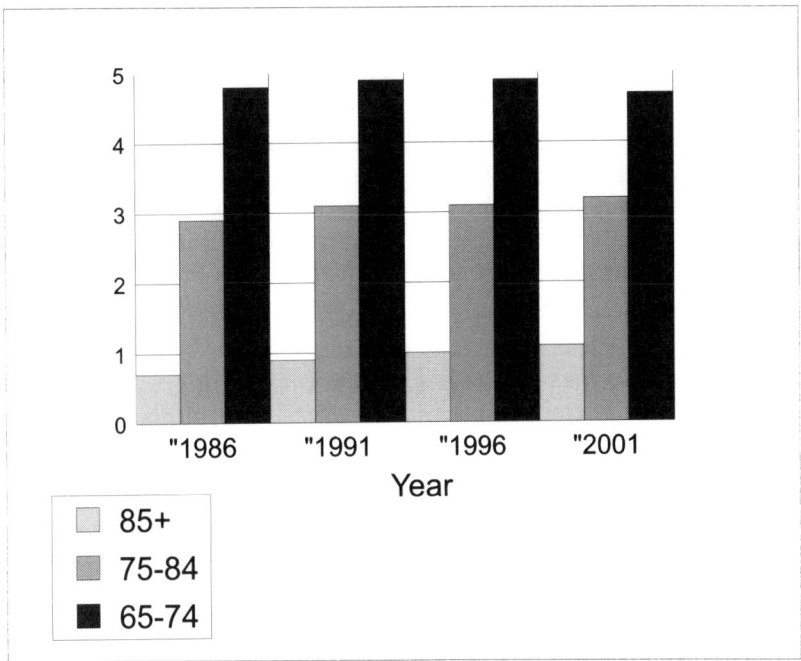

Figure 2.1: Demographic trends in older population. Population trends, 66; National population projections, 1989, HMSO, London

Pathology

ATD, multi-infarct dementia (MID), and Lewy body type dementia(LBTD) account for about 80% of dementia in younger people and for 95% in the elderly. Pathologically there are differences between them.

The pathological changes in dementia have been classified into two groups, one typical of ATD and one with areas of brain softening and infarction which are known as vascular dementias. The term MID has been used to describe the mechanism whereby vascular dementia is produced, but other pathogenic mechanisms may be as important. The terms MID and vascular dementia should not be used synonomously (Amar and Wilcock, 1996).

Pathology of ATD

In ATD the **cerebral hemispheres** demonstrate a marked shrinkage in size and weight and increase in ventricular size, particularly in the young. This shrinkage occurs mainly in the cortex and grey matter with the parietal, temporal and frontal lobes suffering most damage. The hippocampal damage is responsible for disturbances in recent memory recall. Microscopically there are characteristic findings of **senile plaques** and **neurofibrillary tangles**. ATD is not caused by arterial sclerosis.

Senile plaques: These consist of degenerate nerve endings and the abnormal protein beta-amyloid. They are present in greatest number where there is the most brain shrinkage and the number present is proportional to the degree of intellectual deterioration. The formation of amyloid is a major pathological factor in ATD.

Neurofibrillary tangles: These occur at the ends of neurones in affected areas and are possibly the remains of damaged parts of neurones. They are associated with the loss of enzymes involved in neurotransmitter production, particularly acetylcholine.

Damaged neurones: These interfere with neurotransmission. Enzymes related to acetylcholine are greatly reduced in ATD, especially in the hippocampus. Noradrenaline and 5-hydroxytryptamine (5-HT) are also affected, but to a lesser degree, as is the transmitter gamma-aminobutyric acid (GABA). Much of the cerebral nerve damage appears to occur in sub-cortical nuclei in the centre of cerebral hemispheres. Possible mechanisms which may be involved in neuronal death are illustrated in Figure 2.2.

Summary of ATD pathology:

- shrinkage and enlarged ventricles of temporal, parietal and frontal lobes of cerebral hemispheres
- senile plaques; shrinkage and cell loss in the grey matter of the cerebral hemispheres
- neurofibrillary tangles
- loss of the enzymes needed for neurotransmission within the neurones of the cerebral hemispheres
- loss of neurotransmission at the nerve endings in the cerebral cortex.

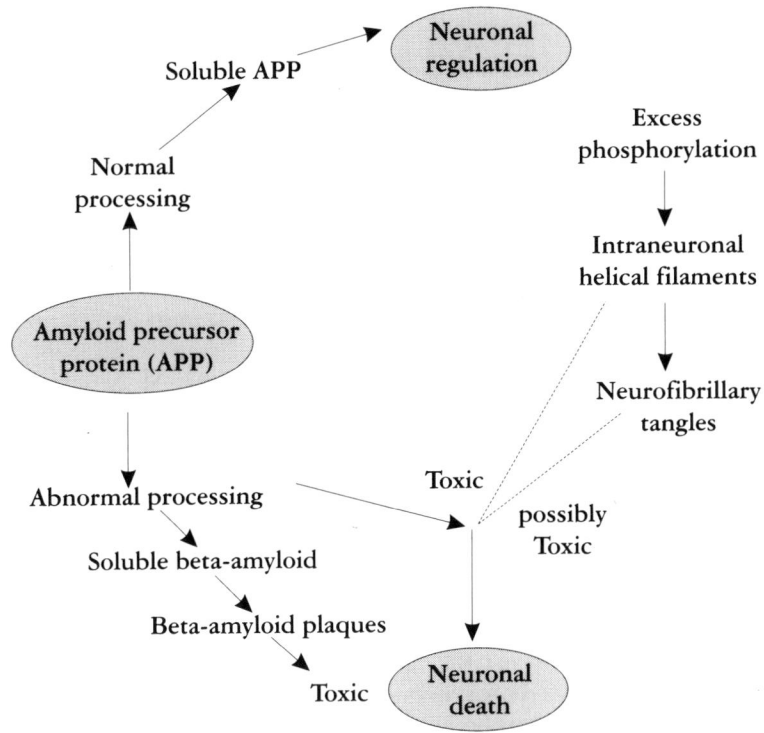

Figure 2.2: Possible mechanisms involved in neuronal death

Aetiology of ATD

It was not until 1993–94 that researchers agreed that ATD had a heterogeneous aetiology that shared the same clinical (behavioural and cognitive) presentation. Recent research suggests that different pathogenic pathways lead to a similar pathological end-point (Shua-Haim, 1996).

ATD is a disorder of specific neurones, especially those that produce acetylcholine. It affects particular cell bodies in the subcortical nuclei, causing a failure of neurotransmission at the axon ends at cortical synapses with a resultant decline in cerebral function. The basic damage may be sustained at the nerve endings where the plaques and tangles are situated, but this has not been confirmed by research. Damage to the nerve cells and the brain may be caused by specific nerve poisons or an increased vulnerability of the cells to ageing. Lead and aluminium are known to damage nerve cells.

Aluminium deposits have been demonstrated in the core of the senile plaques commonly seen in ATD patients. Such deposits may arise from the ingestion of excess dietary aluminium but could well be due to a failure of the mechanisms that normally protect the brain from circulatory aluminium. Ingested aluminium accumulates more in nerve cells already containing the neurofibrillary tangles — the hallmark of all ATDs. Food stored in cans or cooked in aluminium pots and certain drugs, such as antacids, are sources of environmental aluminium. However, no causative links with ingested aluminium and dementia have been substantiated.

ATD is believed to result from a variety of genetic and environmental factors which initiate a cascade of processes that result in brain damage and the symptoms of dementia.

Although much remains unknown about the cause of ATD, it is known that the syndrome predominantly affects older people, is strongly associated with Down's syndrome and there is a marked hereditary factor in a few families.

Genetic causes

There is a genetic basis for the rare familial ATD which is usually of early onset and is passed on as a dominant condition. Familial ATD is a condition in which members of affected families have a higher risk of developing the symptoms of dementia than the rest of the population. Mutations on chromosome 21 have been identified. Mutation in the amyloid precursor protein (APP) gene causes either an increase or a subtle change in the type of **beta-amyloid protein** formed. The assumption is that abnormal metabolism of the beta-amyloid precursor protein is central to the causation of ATD (Kist and Hastie, 1994).

Beta-amyloid protein aggregates to form the thread-like fibrils which accumulate in senile plaques and around blood vessels. It is thought by many researchers to be a control factor in the cause and progression of attend, and its overproduction appears to be an important risk factor for the disease. It may cause cell damage or alter vulnerabilityof cells so that they can be damaged by another process. Other genetic link studies have demonstrated an association between late onset familial ATD and chromosome 19 (Tobianski, 1993) and between early onset familial ATD and chromosome 14. The size of the cortical area affected by beta-amyloid deposition is important in the clinical manifestation of dementia and supports the possibility that beta-amyloid is central to the aetiology of ATD (*Lancet*, 1995).

The role of apoliproteins

Recent research (Corder *et al*, 1993) has demonstrated that the common form of ATD is related to the inheritance of apoliprotein E (apo E). This protein is involved in transporting lipids around the body. It also occurs in the brain where it may be involved in the repair of damaged nerve endings (Poirier *et al*, 1993).

People usually inherit apoliproteins (apo) E3 but can inherit E3 and E4 forms. Inheritance of apo E4 increases the risk of developing ATD fourfold. If the inheritance comes from both parents there is a further increase in risk (Rubinsztein, 1995).

However, inheriting the gene for apo E4 is neither sufficient or necessary for the development of the disease as individuals inheriting apo4 from both parents can remain mentally well throughout life. Half of those who get ATD do not have a copy of the apo E4 gene.

Apo E4 binds more rapidly than its associates to beta-amyloid which may result in increased deposits of amyloid in senile plaques. Inheritance of apo E2 reduces the risk of developing ATD (Rossor, 1993).

Although the apo E4 allele is associated with ATD a preventive strategy for the disease remains a distant goal (Elon, 1996). A full understanding of the pathogenesis of attend remains elusive.

Neurotransmitter deficit

The enzyme involved in the synthesis of acetylcholine is much reduced in the brains of ATD patients and a link has been shown between acetylcholine production and the severity of the dementia. Acetylcholine is a key neurotransmitter in cell-to-cell signalling in the central nervous system — a chemical messenger in the learning and memory processes. The possibility of acetylcholine replacement therapy is a promising treatment for the disease or at least for improving memory. Recent therapeutic advances involve drugs that increase normal levels of acetylcholine by inhibiting the enzyme responsible for breaking it down.

Causes of Dementia

Over 70 causes of dementia have been recognised. The more common ones are:

Primary cerebral degeneration:	Alzheimer's disease (ATD) Parkinson's disease (PD) Lewy body type dementia (LBTD) Huntington's disease
Cerebrovascular disease:	Multi-infarct dementia (MID) (corticovascular dementia) Binswanger's disease (subcortical vascular dementia)
Cerebral infections:	Syphilis, meningitis and human immunodeficiency virus (HIV) infection resulting in acquired-immune deficiency syndrome (AIDS)
Inflammatory systemic disease:	Multiple sclerosis and systemic lupus erythematosus
Trauma and anoxia:	Resulting from brain injury
Toxic causes:	Alcohol and drugs
Metabolic causes:	Hypothyroidism, hypoglycaemia and chronic hepatic and renal problems
Nutritional causes:	Vitamin B_{12} deficiency and malabsorption syndrome.

A useful mnemonic for remembering causes is 'Mama's bitten dad' if causes are tabulated as shown as shown on the following page.

M	Multi-infarct dementia	B	B₁₂ deficiency	D	Drugs
A	Alzheimer's disease	I	Infection	A	All other causes
M	Mixed	T	Trauma	D	Depression
A	Alcoholism	T	Tumour		
S	Subcortical dementia	E	Endocrine		
		N	Normal pressure hydro-cephalus		

Vascular dementias

These are probably the second commonest cause of dementia. Symptomatic stroke increases the risk of developing dementia ninefold.

There appear to be several pathological types of vascular condition, leading to variations in the clinical presentation of dementia. These include MID and single, strategically placed strokes in specific subcortical areas. *Binswanger's disease* and lacunar dementia are still the subjects of research. The former is rare and connected with arterial sclerosis and high blood pressure.

Vascular dementia may be caused by:
- multiple infarcts
- white matter ischaemia
- a strategically placed infarct.

Vascular dementia has been classified into:
- acute onset
- MID
- sub-cortical (WHO, 1993).

Multi-infarct dementia

- MID results from multiple tiny infarcts in the cerebrum and deeper areas of the brain
- the sum total of the foci correlate with the degree of intellectual impairment
- brain damage is patchy although extensive.

In 20–30% of patients with dementia the main cause is arterial disease (vascular dementia). These individuals usually show evidence of generalised arteriosclerosis. However, it is not narrowing of the vessels with reduction in blood flow that damages the nerve cells in MID. In this condition there are multiple tiny foci of damage (ie. infarcts) in the cerebrum and deeper areas of the brain resulting from obstruction of the local blood supply by a small stroke due to emboli or thrombosis. The combination of many small strokes produces MID and explains the irregular progression of this type of dementia over time. The sum total of all the areas of cerebral softening correlate with the degree of intellectual impairment.

Damage to the brain is patchy although widespread. Extensive areas of the cortex can work normally. The cause of death in this type of dementia is frequently another feature of generalised arterial sclerosis, such as coronary artery thrombosis.

Many people with dementia appear to have pathological evidence of ATD and, classic MID. The relative proportions are difficult to determine and are only of practical relevance in attempts to estimate the rate of decline in affected patients. At present, the only distinction to be drawn is that between classic MID and clear-cut ATD.

Diffuse Lewy body type dementia

Physicians have long identified a type of dementia with features of ATD but with a very variable temporal clinical presentation. It has now been identified as a separate pathological entity. Genetically, apo E4 is overrepresented in patients with a Lewy body variant of dementia.

Lewy bodies appear in the cytoplasm of neurones as pink-staining structures. These features are found on postmortem examination in many cases of dementia, particularly when associated with Parkinson's disease (PD). It is not uncommon for people to suffer from PD and AD. In PD there is a loss of nerve cells and large numbers of Lewy bodies in the pigmented nuclei of the brainstem.

Researchers now recognise that a considerable number of dementia patients — possibly 20% (McKeith et al, 1994) — have senile plaques in their cerebral cortex, but very few neurofibrillary tangles. Instead there are Lewy bodies and the disorder is known as Lewy body type dementia. People with LBTD produce even less acetylcholine than those with ATD but in their case the receptors for acetylcholine are preserved. This preservation is probably related to the lack of neurofibrillary tangles that result in receptor loss in ATD. LBTD patients may in future be candidates for acetylcholine replacement therapy.

Non-ATD dementias

These dementias are often called preventable senility (Hachinski, 1992) as hypertension is a major risk factor.

Aetiology is related to the cause of the generalised arteriosclerosis. Causes are probably multifactorial and include diet, smoking and genetic factors. It is not clear why any particular small cerebral vessel should block, causing infarction and cell death.

Treatable causes of dementia

Vitamin deficiencies

Vitamin B_{12} and folic acid deficiencies can result in the development of dementia which is reversible if treated with appropriate medication. Behavioural and memory changes predominate in presentation. Long tract signs, such as peripheral neuropathy and megaloblastic anaemia, may be present. Vitamin B_{12} substitution must be instituted early before irreversible damage has occurred.

Normal pressure hydrocephalus

This condition tends to occur in younger people, and results in dementia where the flow of cerebrospinal fluid inside the brain is obstructed transiently or partially. Normal pressure hydrocephalus can occur after meningitis, neurosurgery or brain injury, causing the ventricles of the brain to swell and the brain substance to become damaged or shrink.

Endocrine disorders

Thyroid and parathyroid disorders can cause dementia. Hypothyroidism is most commonly implicated, causing a dementia that is treatable and reversible.

Tumours

Primary and secondary tumours can result in dementia, often as a later manifestation of the disease.

Infections

Historically syphilis has been a prime cause of dementia. General paralysis of the insane (GPI) usually starts 10–20 years after the initial infection, if that was untreated. GPI is treatable if an antibiotic is given before brain damage becomes severe.

Other causes of dementia

Down's syndrome

People with Down's syndrome are now living longer and almost always develop Alzheimer-type brain changes by middle age. Those with Down's syndrome, which is caused by an abnormality of chromosome 21, develop typical pathological changes of ATD with classic neurotransmitter losses in their brains if they live long enough (Holland, 1994).

Repetitive head injuries

Repeated injury to the brain, as occurs in boxing, may ultimately result in generalised impairment of the cerebral function. Subdural haematoma can also cause dementia.

HIV infection and AIDS

HIV enters the brain and can be a cause of AIDS related dementia which advances quickly to death. It is common in younger patients, among whom there is likely to be a continued increase in the number of sufferers (Navia, 1994).

TB, meningitis, syphilis, toxoplasmosis and encephalitis can all result in dementia.

Creutzfeldt-Jakob disease (CJD) is a rare and rapidly progressive dementia believed to be caused by a slow-acting infectious agent called a 'prion'. A prion is made up only of protein and reproduces by using the cell's own genes, unlike a virus. It has gained recent prominence through its link to bovine spongiform encephalopathy (BSE) in cows.

CJD is the most common clinicopathological sub.type of the transmissable spongiform encephalopathies which occur in inherited, acquired and sporadic form. 86% of human prior disease occurs as a randomly distributed illness of unknown cause — sporadic CJD. The annual incidence is about one per million with onset at 65 years of age and older.

Classically, CJD presents as a rapidly progressive dementia with myoclonus progressing rapidly to akinetic mutism and death. Within 3-4 months most patients have charteristic electro-encephalograms (EEG).

A new variant of CJD linked to BSE appears to have occurred in the UK. It occurs in young people with a clinical course different from sporadic CJD. Behavioural changes are an early feature, ataxia and myoclonus develop with a rapidly progressing dementia leading to death. EEG changes although abnormal are not characteristic of CJD (Will, 1996).

Inflammatory

Multiple sclerosis associated dementia is caused by plaques that develop in the brain's white matter. They differ from the senile plaques of ATD and the grey matter is not affected. There is usually widespread patchy damage and the dementia is often mild.

Neoplastic

Frontal tumours. Multiple metastoses.

Defects in neurotransmitter production

People with Parkinson's disease are more likely to suffer from dementia, with 20% of cases being affected. In this instance, the dementia is thought to be due to a reduction in acetylcholine with affected patients showing pathological evidence of cell death in the nucleus of Meynert. The dementia therefore has similar features to

ATD. People with Huntington's Chorea also suffer from a progressive dementia.

Toxic damage

Dementia can be caused by toxic damage resulting from alcoholism, solvent abuse, aluminium and lead poisoning. Patients with Wilson's disease may develop toxic damage induced dementia when copper levels are not under control.

Korsakoff's syndrome

This occurs in chronic alcoholics. It does not affect the overall functioning of the cerebrum and is not strictly speaking a dementia. However, as in ATD, there appears to be similar reduction in acetylcholine production although it is limited to a small area of the brain. Computerised tomographic scanning has revealed a more generalised shrinking of the brain in chronic alcoholics, which is believed to be a sign of a developing general dementia.

3
The disease process

A progressive disease

The progression of the dementing process over time varies greatly from patient to patient and often from day to day in the individual patient. Some people in the early stages of the illness are adept at hiding symptoms from intrusive observers.

Traditionally, the severity of the disease process has been recorded as mild, moderate or severe, with assessment based largely on cognitive testing. This medical model is of limited value in assessing the need for drug therapy and of little help in practical management or assessment for service provision.

There is a continuum of symptomatology bridging traditional levels of staging. Attempts to demarcate levels of progression of the disease create artificial boundaries and false premises on which to base future management plans. Carr and Marshall (1993), consider staging to be arbitrary and meaningless. The classification of dementia into early, middle and late stages with reference to time can also be misleading, although it is much easier to differentiate early from late presentations of the dementing process.

It is often an assumed that in the late stages of the disease the patient will be hospitalised or in long-term institutional care, whereas in reality many of these individuals live in the community. These arbitrary divisions reveal little about the individual's ability for self-care which is a crucial factor in good primary care management. The terms are frequently used by administrators to define a population of people with dementia occupying long-stay care units in attempts to quantify the degree of deterioration or behavioural problem. The likelihood is that there will be patients at varying levels of the dementing process with differing needs who defy such descriptive group labelling.

A global, holistic approach to the assessment of people exhibiting evidence of a dementing process is recommended, with consideration given to cognition, affect, and physiological, behavioural and medical status of the individual. Functional and self-care skills status are vital factors in obtaining community care. Ability to carry out normal activities of daily living (ADL) and the amount of family or voluntary carer support will largely determine management plans. The emphasis is on appraisal of physical and intellectual function and the potential for continued self-care or self and supported care. Staging of symptomatology should not be the principal factor in overall assessment but it can provide a framework on which to build a diagnostic route to a confirmed diagnosis. However, as Briggs (1993) has noted: 'The medical approach should not exclude social and psychological aspects of management.'

Clinical presentation

Clinical features relate to the progressive damage to the brain, which produces functional brain failure, bringing disinhibition, loss of self-control and behavioural change.

The presenting features will depend on the individual's previous personality, life experience, and premorbid and educational status, with behaviour and response varying from person to person. The needs of the individual patient vary with the progression of the disease and the immediate care support available.

Localised functional deficits occur in:

1. Processing information
2. Receiving information
3. Storing information
4. Speech expression
5. Mobility and coordination.

External evidence of brain deficits varies with the severity of the illness and depends on:

1. Time of day
2. Affective state
3. Fatigue status
4. Audience/onlookers
5. Baseline of educational attainment and cognitive skills.

Loss of control over brain input: Attention may wander or become 'stuck'.

Loss of control over brain output: This results in:

1. Disinhibition in thinking with perseveration and illusion
2. Forward-planning deficits in speech with perseveration and 'stuck' speech
3. Behaviour perseveration, often inappropriate and ritual
4. Disturbance in affect, eg. lability, inappropriateness, catastrophic reaction
5. Immobility, loss of mobility or limitation.

Neurological loss of control: This can result in:

1. Incontinence
2. Fits.

The clinical presentation is very variable and transient in the early stages of the disease. Not all of the deficits will be shown by all of the individuals affected. Other clinical features include memory disability, such as misplacing objects and forgetting familiar names, loss of attention when reading, and poor concentration.

Initially there may be a denial of these symptoms but, eventually they lead to:
- poor work performance
- poor decision taking and making
- social disruption
- decreased ability to manage activities in daily living (ADL).

There is likely to be disorientation in time, place and person with some flattening of affect, which is initially mild but later becomes marked. Depression, apathy, introvertive withdrawal, and emotional lability are all potential symptoms of the disease. These clinical features may be looked at in terms of emotional, cognitive and behavioural changes.

Emotional changes

Emotional changes may feature a shallowness of mood with a swing of affect between apathy and enthusiasm. Emotional responsiveness is variable, and often low-key and inappropriate occurs with the emotive response.

There may be a lack of consideration for others with an

expression of selfishness and self-centredness.

A variable degree of anxiety can be responsible for the emotional and behavioural responses.

Depression can be a response to patients' awareness of the significance of their symptoms. This may be overt or masked and is often missed by GPs and professional and family carers.

In the progressive stages of the illness, patients may display marked irritability and hostility towards carers, with associated aggression.

Cognitive changes

Cognition can be defined as the ability to use and manipulate language, and dependence, memory, state of awareness, language function, visuospatial function and mental tempo. In dementia:

- there is short-term memory impairment with difficulty in recalling new information
- thinking becomes concrete and inflexible
- there is a repetitiveness of speech with perseverance of thoughts and repetitiveness of activities
- language disorders can result in both receptive and expressive dysphasia and speech becomes disordered and fragmented
- there may well be ideas of persecution, delusions and auditory and visual hallucinations.

These latter psychotic features may occur in 30–40% of dementing patients.

Behavioural changes

Behavioural changes include:
- difficulty in carrying out ADL
- inappropriate social behaviour
- social withdrawal
- self-neglect
- emotional disinhibition
- wandering and restlessness
- 'sundowning' and the turning of night into day
- aggression and violence
- disorientation in terms of time, place and people.

In the later stages of the disease, symptoms may include: weight loss resulting from malnutrition and self-neglect, bradykinesis and tremor; and rigidity of muscles in the body, instability, immobility and ultimately incontinence of urine and faeces. Loss of mobility leads to falls, while speech difficulties and thinking disorder bring loss of communication skills and loss of control. Disinhibition can result in socially unacceptable sexual and moral behaviour.

Any significant change in behaviour that is inconsistent with patterns of previous well-established premorbid personality is suggestive of an organic pathology.

Carelessness of speech or dress and easy fatiguability are signs of early organic change. Behavioural disturbance in dementia is at least partly dependent on context. The disturbed behaviour may be an understandable response to the behaviour of others or to personal perceptions of pain or discomfort. Disturbed behaviour can also be precipitated by complex mental state delusions. Behavioural changes may include social withdrawal, abuse of alcohol and sexual aberration.

Other presentations

Dementia may come to the doctor's attention at any point in its development from mild memory loss at one end of the spectrum to major cognitive physical and behavioural deterioration at the other. Clinical features can usefully be considered in terms of the five:

- amnesia
- aphasia
- apraxia
- agnosia
- associated personality and behavioural change (Burns and Hallewell, 1995).

Amnesia

Amnesia is often the first sign noticed by patients and relatives. It may range from forgetting recent events or knowledge to complete disruption of all memory, both recent and remote. The initial problem is failure to commit new information to long-term memory which progresses to failure to retrieve older memories. The effects on the patient are:

- frequent loss of everyday objects
- repeated telephone calls to relatives
- repetition of conversations
- failure to keep appointments.

Aphasia

Nominal aphasia is often an early sign of dementia, with the patient unable to name objects.

Apraxia

Apraxia is the inability to perform coordinated motor tasks although peripheral power and sensations remain intact. This leads to disturbance in ADL which can progress to inability to dress, eat or toilet.

Agnosia

Agnosia is the failure to recognise sensory stimuli although peripheral senses are intact. This often results in inability to recognise the spouse and failure to identify objects and smells.

Personality changes

Characteristically, people with dementia have little or no insight into changes in their personality, but premorbid personality and the quality of relationships with others influence the type of personality change exhibited. Personality change is often accompanied by a loss of social skills, which is initially trivial but becomes progressively more disabling; it is therefore not surprising that the symptomatology includes disorders of mood and affect, with evidence of irritability, anxiety and depression. These are possibly reactions by the patient to an awareness of failing powers.

In dementia, the processes of cognition — perceiving, thinking and remembering, mood, emotion and behaviour — are all disturbed, but the degree of derangement of each component varies from person to person and according to the duration and development of the illness (Cramond, 1969). These presenting clinical features are important considerations in making a diagnosis but if the GP bases the diagnosis solely on these features, an optimal quality of care management for the patient will not be achieved.

In 1968, Blessed *et al* described the changes found in the brains of 50 patients at autopsy. The subjects had shown signs of dementia before death and comparisons and measurements were made to determine the nature of the changes associated with dementia in old age. It was found that the amount of neurological damage did not match the level of signs and symptoms which each individual had displayed. The researchers concluded that dementia could not be explained in purely technical terms and that other factors needed to be considered.

The medical model of treatment should not exclude social and psychological aspects (Briggs, 1993). A holistic view of dementia is endorsed by Kitwood (1988) who views dementia as involving not just neurological impairment but also personality, personal biography, health, social and psychological status. He believes that dementia is an existential plight of persons, not simply a problem to be investigated technically. To this equation should be added consideration of the environment and the actions of others.

This global approach is vital in assessment of the patient with dementia. Another model, drawn from the sociological field, views dementia as a disability, recognising that a major consideration in the incapacity of many people with dementia is the way that health professionals and others relate to them and to interpersonal social interaction. Dementia, then, is not just the patient's problem, but a problem for the professional too. This emphasises the need for the doctor to strive to create a degree of empathy with the patient.

4
Making the diagnosis

Detection and early diagnosis

GPs have been criticised by people with dementia and carers, who feel abandoned by the medical profession (Lewis, 1995). Surveys (Alzheimer's Disease Society [ADS] England, 1995) have shown that 42% of family doctors appear to give no indication of what might be the matter with the dementing patient, on initial consultation. The majority do not carry out memory testing on patients presenting with symptoms of early dementia (ADS, 1993). GPs are known to be poorly motivated to carry out regular structured assessments of longer-term, mentally ill patients (Ledesert and Ritchie, 1994). Data from a major study suggest that the typical patient with Alzheimer-type dementia (ATD) is diagnosed 32 months after symptom onset (Jost and Grossberg, 1995), with a longer delay in people less than 65 years of age.

A multidisciplinary approach to dementia care is still rare in general practice and, in most cases, initial assessment is carried out in a limited fashion by the doctor or social worker (Griffiths, 1988; Hunter and Griffiths, 1988). The NHS and Community Care Act has thrust the social worker to the fore in the provision of services for mentally ill patients; however, there are risks associated with their making an assessment and arranging provision of care if this is based largely on grounds of functional incapacity.

A common concern among clinicians has been the fear that early detection of dementia will merely increase demand on overburdened services (Malcolm, 1993). Lack of early recognition with resultant delay in the provision of services adds to patient and family carers' suffering and results in crisis demands being made on the health professional. Early recognition and diagnosis of the disease with prompt, appropriate advice given to family carers increases awareness of availability of help and decreases stress, apparently without increasing resources (Horowitz, 1985; Philp and Young, 1988). In a typical general practice with a normal proportion of elderly people, two new patients with dementia can be expected each year (Schoenberg et al, 1987).

It is important to recognise dementia early in order to:
- differentiate clinical types

- exclude differential diagnoses
- identify treatable conditions
- facilitate management decisions and avert crises
- advise and support patients and carers
- encourage treatment (Copeland *et al*, 1986).

Advising the person with ATD of the diagnosis

Whether or not to tell the patient newly diagnosed with attend the nature of their illness is still a source of controversy. In America, published guidelines state categorically that the patient should be informed (Post and Whitehouse, 1995), but there is no absolutely right or wrong answer: each doctor and family must make a private and personal decision. Telling the patient requires tact, sensitivity and consideration, and must be accompanied by information about means of coping with the illness.

The affected person and the family should come to understand that:
- ATD is progressive and irreversible
- some symptoms can be treated
- support groups are available
- NHS and social support will be available
- a care plan will be discussed with them.

If a patient is only mildly cognitively impaired and capable of understanding the diagnosis and the implications, withholding the knowledge from him/her is unfair and unethical as the patient is being deprived of the right to know the diagnosis. Not to tell robs the individual of the opportunity to prepare for declining health and indulgence in activities, such as travel, while still able to do so.

In a mildly impaired patient, most doctors emphasise the early status of the disorder and the slow rate of decline. Patients who are severely affected when told the diagnosis are likely to forget the revelation anyway, but telling the facts in front of relatives can have a 'cathartic' effect if there are further secrets being withheld between the relatives.

Pros and cons of telling the patient the diagnosis

Advantages of advising the patient:

- respects the individual's right to know the truth
- provides the patient with the opportunity to seek information and get treatment available
- permits advance planning of financial and personal nature
- presents the opportunity for patients to express their preferences in treatment and to resolve conflicts and wishes for the future before cognitive function declines
- permits the doctor to discuss involvement of partners, eg. in driving
- allows patient and family to access a spiritual adviser while coming to terms with the diagnosis
- allows the patient to participate in counselling and support group intervention which may help to alleviate anger, self-blame, fear and depression.

Disadvantages of advising the patient:

- diagnosis cannot be made with perfect accuracy
- prognosis is difficult to determine
- therapeutic options are limited
- disclosure of diagnosis may precipitate depression, catastrophic reaction and functional decline
- patient may not understand the diagnosis.

Early studies suggesting that the majority of GPs were unaware of dementing patients in their practices have not been supported by more recent work (Philp and Young, 1988; Philp, 1989). On the positive side, GPs in a Scottish study were aware of 58% of their patients with dementia living in the community and 55% of those living in residential and nursing homes (Gordon et al, 1993). However, awareness may be long delayed after the onset of the illness and further delay can occur before diagnosis is confirmed. In one study, in a third of cases it took more than a year for a diagnosis of Alzheimer's disease or other dementia to be confirmed (ADS, 1995). Only 13% of carers of patients with dementia felt they had been given sufficient information at diagnosis concerning the chronic and progressive nature of the disease. However, when considering early presentations of dementia, doctors are dealing with possibilities rather than absolutes; doubts about the accuracy of the diagnosis can dominate management in the early stages of the disease.

There are benefits in seeking early diagnosis of dementia for the patient, for the carer and for the doctor and primary care team.

Those with a dementing illness suffer a progressive loss of intellectual functioning which will ultimately interfere with decision-making and taking. This is not usually an 'all-or-none' process (Rabins and Mace, 1986) but occurs at a variable rate with varying impact on the reasoning process.

Although patients are possibly disorientated in time and place, their ability to make judgments may be unimpaired, which means that in the early phase of a dementing process individuals can still be aware of their current experience and anticipate needs. They should not be denied the right to plan for their future for as long as they can offer rational, reasoned contributions to the management plan.

They must therefore be included in meetings relating to events affecting their declining health (Davis, 1988). It is important that physicians and members of the family respect the competence of the patient. This involvement of patients can, for example, be used to establish powers of attorney over finances and include agreements about the patient's participation in future research (Goldsmith, 1996). This involvement can leave patients feeling that they have some control over their own destinies.

Benefits of early diagnosis for the patient:

- respects the individual's right to know the truth
- affords the opportunity to seek adequate information and treatment
- permits the patient to plan for the future provision of the legal, financial and health care services (Kennedy and Rossor, 1993)
- patients feel that they are getting medical support while they still have insight into the disease (Bloom, 1993)
- awareness of declining function produces greatest stress in patients with recent onset of the disease, and counselling and support are then of considerable value

- enables the patient to receive prompt treatment for concomitant conditions, eg. a current mental disorder such as depression appears to cause unnecessary disability in dementing patients (McLean, 1993)
- permits the patient to resolve past conflicts, eg. family disagreements, and record last wishes and allows access to spiritual adviser.

Benefits of early diagnosis for the carer:

- carers feel that they are getting some medical support at a very traumatic time
- allows the identification of carer stress which may be alleviated or shared by appropriate service input
- provision of early information. Relatives appear to want to be told about a diagnosis of dementia as soon as possible (Kennedy and Rossor, 1993)
- carers view the diagnosis as providing 'a gateway to services' (Jacques, 1992)
- knowledge of the diagnosis provides carers with an explanation for the patient's bizarre behaviour and stops them blaming the patient or themselves
- enables the carer to acknowledge the patient's preferences
- knowledge of the diagnosis can now be shared with the patient.

Benefits of early diagnosis for the doctor:

- early assessment in diagnosis allows forward planning in terms of service provision, respite care and resource management for fundholding practices
- additional early support for the carer in reducing stress may decrease the workload on the family doctor at a later date
- allows early involvement of the primary care team
- permits confirmation of the diagnosis
- treatable conditions can be excluded
- concomitant physical conditions can be treated
- programme of regular reassessments can be constructed
- the opportunity for information and education of patient and

carer such as a programme of patient activity can be given
- patient's preferences based on their life experience can be recorded
- there is the opportunity for preventive action, eg. in reducing the risk of car accidents by enforcing a ban on the patient driving him/herself.

Problems arising from early diagnosis

Resources to meet the patient's needs may be unavailable, and the raised expectations of carer and patient which cannot be met may cause frustration for the doctor and the care team. Patient and carer may also have to live longer with the diagnosis. There is some evidence too that earlier diagnosis brings with it the possibility of earlier institutionalisation (O'Connor, 1993). Early diagnosis may also precipitate depressive illness.

However, full assessment of patients with failing cognitive capacity facilitates the detection and treatment of medical conditions that cause confusion, which can be mistaken for dementia. Drug treatment can also be reviewed (McLean, 1987; Zarit et al, 1985).

Early diagnosis is only of value if it is accurate. Inaccurate diagnosis can be not only misleading but dangerous in terms of unrecognised and untreated concomitant illness. GPs make three kinds of error in diagnosis:

1. Underdiagnosis — where there is failure to recognise the onset of dementia.
2. Overdiagnosis — where a non-dementing illness is diagnosed as dementia (Gordon, 1991; Iliffe, 1992).
3. Misdiagnosis — where cognitive impairment is attributed to a functional psychosis.

It is usually depression which is misdiagnosed. The diagnosis of dementia can be difficult as the symptoms can be diverse and non-specific. It is particularly difficult in the early stages, when symptoms resemble age-associated memory changes. All three situations have their dangers: overdiagnosis can lead to a possibly treatable illness being missed; misdiagnosis may result in a dementing illness being diagnosed as depression, for example, and being mistreated; and underdiagnosis where the patient fails to receive appropriate management and attention for a dementing process.

In the absence of a definitive test for dementia, accurate diagnosis depends largely on longitudinal assessments of a variety of areas of physiological and cognitive functioning. GPs tend to overdiagnose when they use formal testing devices to assess cognitive function (O'Connor, 1993). Sadly, diagnostic tools such as measuring scales and cognitive assessment tests are rarely used in daily practice.

Some of the reluctance to use diagnostic screens, such as formal cognitive tests may be due to fear of insulting the patient or causing distress. The same researcher found no evidence however to suggest that patients were actually distressed by the use of such testing methods. Although they are insufficient in themselves to establish a firm diagnosis, cognitive tests can provide valuable information and, with repetition, help to identify patients with a dementing process.

GP detection rate for dementia

The poor rate of detection of dementia by GPs has been attributed to:

1. Undergraduate and postgraduate inadequacies in training. GPs who have been long qualified are more likely to assume that cognitive decline is an inevitable part of ageing (Iliffe, 1994).
2. Disinterest, often generated by a fear of increased workload or feelings of therapeutic inadequacy.
3. A nihilistic approach to dementia management (Archibald, 1996).
4. A lack of assessment protocols.
5. Legitimate difficulties in making a firm diagnosis.
6. Failure of patients to present with memory complaints and failure of family members to bring behavioural problems and memory changes to the GP's attention. Only a quarter of those caring for mildly impaired relatives and two-fifths of those caring for moderately impaired relatives had raised the subject of dementia with their GPs (O'Connor *et al*, 1988).
7. Ageist attitudes to management of a condition found primarily in the elderly.

A survey of GPs' ability to recognise mild dementia as a diagnostic possibility found that half the cases were identified (O'Connor et al, 1988) despite an absence of formal tests of orientation and memory. This suggests that if they were regularly to apply brief cognitive tests, which take only a couple of minutes, and question relatives about changes in memory, intellect and behaviour, GPs' diagnostic accuracy would improve considerably. As GPs see relatively few patients with dementia, 'performance anxiety' in assessment, diagnosis and referral to specialists can occur (O'Hanlon, 1987). In an Australian survey of GPs, inadequate knowledge or expertise was common, with doctors often feeling at a loss when patients and carers asked about latest treatment (Brodaty et al, 1994).

Improving diagnostic skills

The need for additional training for GPs has been recognised (Alzheimer's Disease Society, 1995). Lack of training has resulted in a lack of confidence on the part of GPs in making a firm diagnosis. Apart from having to deal with intrinsic difficulties inherent in the diagnosis of dementia, the GP is also more vulnerable to irrational decision-making procedures because of external pressures from caregivers and socio-economic considerations (Ledesert and Ritchie, 1994).

GPs need to be aware that the patient is unlikely to bring cognitive failings directly to the doctor's attention and that carers in the family tend to minimise them until such failings are well established in the later stages of the disorder.

Training should include the use of a standardised assessment protocol and standardised screening instruments, such as the mini-mental state examination (MMSE) and abbreviated mental test (AMT), to determine impairment. Infrequent use of screening tests and recourse to standardised diagnostic criteria appear to be largely a result of GPs' belief that they are unsuitable for clinical practice (Somerfield et al, 1991); however, in some practices they are used routinely by doctors and nurses (McIntosh et al, 1988).

The use of depression rating scales such as the Geriatric Depression Scale (Yesavage and Brink, 1983) or Brief Assessment of Depression Schedule (BASDEC) cards can also help to exclude depression in the differential diagnosis.

A willingness to organise a magnetic resonance imaging (MRI) scan, or refer a patient for MRI scan via a consultant, in early dementia cases is also essential. Training may also change attitudes and sharpen diagnostic skills. Both GPs and families appear to have low expectations of what general practice has to offer dementing elderly people (O'Connor et al, 1988). Nihilistic management, where it is assumed that dementia inevitably leads to gross behavioural disturbance, immobility, incontinence and incoherence, will encourage negative reactions in doctor and carer. Many of those with dementia never reach this advanced state, and liaison with relatives and supportive management can make early intervention satisfying for doctor, patient and carer.

Assessment procedures

Empathic support and advice to families are important during early investigations when the diagnosis of dementia, although not corroborated, may be feared by patient and carer. An understanding of pressures on the carer will be appreciated, and even at this early stage supportive intervention may be beneficial. In both diagnosis and supportive management, GPs and the primary care team have a crucial role which demands a knowledge of available non-medical supportive services and links with the social services. A caring GP should be fully aware of the existence, availability and role of local memory clinics and institutional support services if assessment and earlier diagnosis of the disease are to be beneficial. The availability of support services can vary in different geographical areas.

There is a paramount need for the GP to take the initiative if dementing patients are to be identified earlier and the detection rate is to improve. The advent of annual geriatric screening for people over 75 years of age offers an ideal opportunity for screen- ing for dementia. However, this contractual obligation has been running for several years, with scant evidence of standardisation of procedures, measuring instruments and data collection. Assessment can be carried out by the doctor, community nurse, health visitor or lay helper and assessment programmes vary from simple questionnaires without intermittent surveillance, to comprehensive longitudinal scoring systems based on regular intervention. Few of these have been validated and the majority do not include a memory test. Unfortunately, once accumulated, the data appear to attract little attention and scant analysis and are rarely used in any rolling programme of surveillance (Wilkieson et al, 1996).

The procedure has been welcomed by patients (McIntosh, 1993;

Chew et al, 1994). In the absence of proper precautions, however, the process of assessment can cause psychological distress to both patient and carer in terms of false reassurance, failure to provide promised support and concern over further potential investigations. It brings to the patient an added awareness of likely morbidity and mortality and the intervention can disturb the individual's perception of personal health (McIntosh, 1994). The health professional should be aware of the potential impact of assessment on the patient and endeavour to negate adverse effects by adequate explanation, service provision and follow-up.

Medical, physical and psychiatric problems that are common in elderly people are just as common in elderly people with dementia. Symptoms due to cardiac conditions, arthritis and simple infections can cause as much distress to the patient with dementia as they do to the mentally intact, but are more easily missed when the patient has communication problems. Good, general examination and regular reassessment are therefore essential for people with dementia.

This calls for a medical, physical, psychological and social assessment protocol incorporating a comprehensive assessment check list which can be used both in annual geriatric assessment and in more frequent assessments on patients. Several of these have been validated. One is the over 75 year old assessment protocol used in my own practice for many years. It includes a memory-rating scale and functional assessment chart (see Appendix 4) (McIntosh, 1990; Young and Chamove, 1989). The patient with dementia merits a full physical check-over at initial presentation and at regular intervals thereafter. Ascertaining functional status and intellectual performance is of vital importance. If this is not carried out there can be only limited appreciation of the patient's needs. A functional check of this nature demands a comprehensive review of activities of daily living (ADL). This involves asking the following questions. Is the patient:

1. Coping with routine tasks ADL?
2. Safe in the confines of the home environment?
3. Disoriented in time and place?
4. Showing overt anxiety or depression?
5. Having obvious memory lapses?

The ability to carry out ADL is crucial for patients who are to be cared for in the home setting. Failure to carry out these activities will often

mean institutionalisation. ADL involves:
- dressing
- self-care
- continence
- cooking skills
- shopping abilities
- financial abilities
- maintenance of social contacts.

These reviews are frequently made by a health visitor or occupational therapist and are not necessarily the remit of the doctor, but they have to be performed before an assessment can be made of the patient's needs. Comprehensive assessment of the dementing patient is needed not only for diagnostic purposes but is also of crucial importance in defining the needs of patient and carer and in establishing appropriate support systems for both.

In a Forth Valley Health Board study, 25 different assessment protocols in geriatric assessment were used by 49 practices and the majority of these carried no cognitive assessment instrument (Wilkieson *et al*, 1996). It therefore appears likely that across the UK a cognitive screening test for dementia is not routinely incorporated in many geriatric assessment questionnaires. High scores in the AMT and the MMSE suggest strongly that a dementing process may be present and further cognitive assessment is indicated. A memory test such as the AMT or MMSE should be included (Clarke *et al*, 1991) in routine assessments.

Qualitative contractual geriatric assessment should identify the majority of patients in the early stage of dementia. Realistically, with many practices operating on an opportunistic contact basis, the majority of new patients are likely to be picked up if a simple cognitive assessment is performed at this consultation. A patient presenting with a syndrome of memory difficulties, behaviour problems and change in mental faculties should alert the GP to the need for further investigation and a potential diagnosis of dementia. In the diagnostic process it is important to measure the patient's functioning against the standard of what he/she was able to do in the past in terms of skills, education and achievement. This comparative measure is dependent upon historic details obtained from patient and carer.

Making the diagnosis

Standardised assessment procedures and management responses help to:
1. Confirm diagnosis
2. Exclude differential diagnoses and treatable conditions
3. Assess the needs of patient and carer
4. Create a management plan
5. Organise reassessment.

Essential elements in making the diagnosis

These may be summarised as follows:
1. Full history from the patient
2. A history from a close relative or caring carer or close friend
3. Objective assessment of cognitive capacity including the use of a screening instrument
4. A full medical and functional examination
5. Appropriate investigations.
6. Appropriate referral.

History taking

In taking a history an eye witness account is essential. The length of the history may help to separate dementia from delirium.

Visual and tactile hallucinations:	Tend to indicate delirium
Auditory hallucinations:	Usually indicate psychosis
Olfactory hallucinations:	May indicate epilepsy or tumour

A drug and alcohol history is important and should include a history from carers. It should include over-the-counter drugs and other family members' drugs. Remember that even sweet old ladies can have an alcohol problem!

Head injury is often overlooked unless it is specifically asked about.

There are no completely satisfactory diagnostic criteria which allow a clear diagnosis of depression to be made in people with dementia. Patients should always be asked about loss of interest, early morning wakening, decreased appetite and suicidal thoughts as well as directly about their mood. Nevertheless, other factors such as the general demeanour of the patient may be sufficient to give a clue to the presence of depression.

In the early stages, patients may be able to give a history of memory loss and difficulties in decision-making and concentration. However, in Alzheimer's disease it is often family members who are aware of the gradual development of forgetfulness, with repetition and perseveration of speech and problems with decision- making. Evidence of a gradual onset of symptoms points towards Alzheimer's disease whereas a history of a sudden onset of difficulties is more likely to be associated with stroke and multi-infarct dementia. Recent onset also separates out acute confusional states. The history should identify problems with memory, language, abstract thinking, judgmental problems, difficulties in decision-taking, motor skill loss, personality change, delusional ideas and behavioural problems.

This is an opportunity to discover patients' reactions and attitudes to their illness. Are things from the patient's past now affecting judgment, dependence, outlook? Is there insight, apathy, indifference, frustration? A careful history may well elucidate the different types of dementia. Their recognition may have an effect on later management as new drugs appear to work best in certain types of disorder.

History from the carer

Most patients with moderate or severe dementia are cared for in the community by spouse or children (Twigg, 1992). Family members are likely to be the first to draw attention to the disease process experienced by the relative. They are likely to reveal most information about the individual's current and past status and a history of both should be sought, although the veracity of this history may be affected by the carer's response to the situation. Neighbours and servcice carers such as home helps, meals on wheels providers and other health professionals will also provide confirmatory information that may help to establish the diagnosis.

Disturbed behaviour and relationships are poorly tolerated by caregivers (Levin *et al*, 1989) and are more likely to be reported. This may distort the global picture of the patient's health status and personhood which the history taker is endeavouring to establish. History should encompass the patient's previous personality, education, achievements, interests and social function to provide a baseline on which to measure intellectual and functional decline. This is also the opportunity to explore professional or voluntary carers' expectations, feelings and attitudes to the illness, their duties, future involvement and the quality of the relationships between them and the patient. Indifferent or antagonistic attitudes may bias preferred information and hidden agendas should be considered.

Objective assessment of cognitive ability

Very simple patient questioning may point towards memory losses: registration and recall of a name and address may prove a difficult task even at an early stage in the disease process. Prompts to register and recall three unrelated words, eg. orange, wall and pound, may demonstrate memory deficit and suggest the need for more formal testing and screening tests. However, simple tests such as the MMSE or the ABT take only a few minutes to perform and can provide useful information about cognitive state, especially if repeated at intervals. High scores have to be interpreted with caution and previous educational skills have to be taken into consideration. High scores on these tests point towards and support other evidence of a dementing process. They can easily be added to a general geriatric assessment protocol. They could equally be used by other members of the primary care team. Fears by practitioners that they might embarrass their patients or meet with poor compliance are not grounded in fact (see Appendixes 1 and 5 for examples).

> Asking patients about their memory and concentration can provide a useful lead to the need for a formal screening test, to which most people will agree, if encouraged and reassured that it is a routine exercise in the practice. Simple memory tests should be used by GPs when screening patients for evidence of dementia.

The medical examination

The initial clinical examination should be meticulous as often, in the later stages, little information can be obtained from the patient. Diagnosis depends on the confirmation of the presence of dementia and the exclusion of other possible causes of cognitive disability. Evidence should be sought for the **existence of systemic diseases** which may be exacerbating the dementia and for other primary causes of cognitive impairment. **Focal neurological signs,** and signs and symptoms of thyroid disorder, anaemia, neoplasia, infection, malnutrition, arteriosclerotic disease, hepatic and renal disease and chronic alcoholism, for example, should be identified. The effects of **acute confusional states and depression** have to be kept in mind. The diagnosis is made on clinical grounds. Accuracy of diagnosis increases when standardised assessment criteria are applied (McKhann, 1984). Special attention should be given to the detection of vascular risk factors such as hypertension, heart disease and diabetes and the causes of thromboembolism.

Brain biopsy

The definitive diagnosis of Alzheimer's disease requires neuropathological confirmation and is usually only possible at Postmortem. Other less intensive investigations can lend support to the diagnosis.

Review of drug medication

Polypharmacy is frequently a cause of toxic confusion in elderly people. For reasons of toxicity, compliance and interaction, it is important that drug use should be reviewed at regular intervals and drug medication reduced to a minimum — particularly when psychotropic medication is being considered. The adverse effects of alcohol and hypnotics must be kept in mind if antipsychotic drug use is contemplated. Tricyclic antidepressants may be indicated for depression but they often cause problems when combined with antipsychotic medication. Antipsychotics also exacerbate move- ment disorder when used in Parkinson's disease and usually cause worsening of symptoms and confusion in patients with Lewy body type dementia.

Blood investigations

Routine **blood and biochemical testing** can be carried out at initial presentation or on a repeat visit. Such tests will primarily rule out other potentially treatable causes of dementia and identify other pathologies influencing the symptoms. Routine blood tests should include:

Full blood count	Haemoglobin
ESR and folic acid levels	Thyroid function
Vitamin B_{12} status	Syphilitic serology

Full blood count	Anaemia increases confusion. A raised white count may indicate infection. A raised mean corpuscular volume (MCV) may indicate vitamin B_{12}/folate deficiency or chronic alcohol consumption.
Erythrocyte sedimentation rate (ESR)	An elevated ESR suggests more than simple dementia.
Glucose	May detect hypoglycaemia.
Urea and electrolytes	Will detect renal failure, the commonest cause being drugs.
Liver function tests	May suggest alcohol abuse, cardiac failure or hepatic secondaries.
Vitamin B_{12} & folate	Deficiencies of these are a cause of reversible dementia.
Syphilitic serology	Syphilis is probably worth treating if present.
Urine dipstick test (including leucocytes)	Urinary tract infections are common.

Depending upon the presence of other clincial signs, the following investigations may be indicated:

Bone screen	Hyperparathyroidism is associated with confusion.
Sputum culture/cytology	If productive cough is a feature.
ECG	If chest pain or cardiac failure is a feature.

Other investigations

Urine should also be tested for glucose and protein and sent for culture and sensitivity testing, particularly if there is evidence of urinary incontinence. Urinary tract infection is a frequent cause of confusion in the elderly.

Weight should be measured to exclude problems due to malnutrition and be reviewed regularly.

Radiological investigations

Chest X-ray: This may be indicated if chest infection or neoplasia is suspected. It is the most sensitive way to diagnose congestive cardiac failure which, if untreated, will aggravate dementia (Kist and Hastie, 1995).

Computerised tomography (CT): CT scans are recognised as being a widely available and applicable brain imaging technique to exclude causes of dementia other than ATD. It may show characteristic patterns suggestive of Alzheimer's disease. It detects enlargement of the cerebral ventricles and widening of the Sulci — a possible indication of degenerative brain disease. Its use can exclude conditions such as hydrocephalus and space-occupying lesions. CT scan is helpful in defining the extent of cerebrovascular disease and confirming normal pressure hydrocephalus (NPH). It will also show subdural haematomas and infarcts. Except where NPH or subdural haematoma is suspected on clinical grounds, CT scan is unlikely to alter management. It can be an expensive procedure and is not routinely indicated in patients aged over 75 when the clinical picture is equivocally one of dementia. CT requires patients to remain still for 15 minutes during the procedure and this is often beyond the capabilities of older people with dementia.

Magnetic resonance imaging: MRI scans are more sensitive than CT scans because of higher resolution. They are useful in the identification of ischaemic lesions and can help to detect ATD at an early stage. Another new investigative procedure, **positron emission tomography** (PET), is available in a few areas of the UK. It can show a characteristic profile for ATD in comparison with other types of dementia. It identifies a global reduction in cerebral metabolism, particularly prominent in the parietal and temporal lobes of ATD patients. PET can measure the function of brain cells by analysing the brain's ability to use glucose. In ATD the affected parts of the brain are shown to be non-functioning.

Single photon emission computerised tomography (SPECT): This technique has some promise for the future in elucidating the type of dementia present. A radio-active labelled marker produces images of cerebral blood flow. In infarction there is complete absence of blood from the area because of tissue death, whereas in ATD there is reduced blood flow. SPECT scan may show early changes of temporoparietal hypometabolism in ATD before neuropsychological deficits become apparent (Kist and Hastie, 1995). Patients with vascular dementia tend to show asymmetrical patches of reduced blood flow.

Predictive genetic testing:

Apolipoprotein E4 allele is associated with a dose-dependent risk for late onset ATD and in future a genetic test may have predictive value as to the likely onset of ATD (Rubinsztein, 1995).

Onward referral of the patient

Access to investigations, resources, consultants and institutions varies markedly across the UK and even between neighbouring areas. The advent of fund-holding practice has also further complicated the management scene. Suspicion of a diagnosis of dementia should not automatically prompt a referral to hospital consultant or department. In many cases there may not be a clearly delineated route for referral: in different areas, geriatricians, psychogeriatricians, psychiatrists and GPs may accept responsibility for people with dementia. The caring GP should be prepared to follow the guidelines recommended in this chapter before considering consultant referral.

The general principles that guide GPs in the management of most of their patients should apply to patients with cognitive losses also. They are entitled to the work-up and investigations which can be organised and monitored within the practice and to onward referral where appropriate. The support of all the members of the care team can be utilised and recourse made to further investigation or consultant opinion and management only if involvement passes beyond the skills of the primary care team. It is equally important, however, that ageist attitudes and therapeutic nihilism do not prevent the patient being referred for investigations, which may clearly determine the existence or progression of the disease or exclude treatable or reversible causes of illness that mimics dementia.

Earlier identification and diagnosis of dementing syndromes may well mean that more patients will be referred in future. The advent of new investigative procedures such as MRI and predictive genetic testing may also increase referrals as access to these procedures can often only be obtained via a consultant. With many clinicians potentially involved, patients can easily fall between stools and receive poor treatment. This is a consideration that the GP should keep in mind (Smith, 1995) to ensure optimal provision of support and facilities.

Referral to a hospital consultant: This may be appropriate in order to:

1. Obtain diagnosis of an early dementing syndrome
2. Confirm that a confounding disease is not causing a dementa-like syndrome
3. Detect treatable and reversible causes
4. Request further investigations, such as MRI scans
5. Obtain specialist assessment of management
6. Acquire advice on appropriate drug therapy for behavioural problems
7. Access other specialist services
8. Organise respite care and long-stay placement
9. Access a memory clinic.

Referral to social services: Under the provisions of the 1992 Community Care Act, the social services now have a vital part to play

in the long-term care of people with dementia. Early referral of such people for assessment by social services may circumvent the long wait for attention by patients who are in urgent need of these services.
In response to medical and social referrals, one might expect:
1. Reports of further investigations, such as CT
2. The exclusion of treatable causes
3. Confirmation of diagnosis
4. A mutually agreed management plan embracing medical, functional and social needs
5. In-depth discussion with family and support carers
6. Consideration of appropriate drug therapy
7. Consideration of long-term placement if and when the need arises
8. A list of involved organisations.

Memory clinics

Memory clinics have recently appeared on the British scene. They are still relatively few in number, but can be a real boon for the GP with one in the local area, in the assessment of a patient with memory loss. Access to the clinic is usually arranged by the GP — once again demonstrating the key role that he/she has to play in helping patients with dementia.
The objectives of memory clinics are to:
- provide a comprehensive, integrated, diagnostic resource for people with pronounced memory problems
- identify patients with dementia as early as possible
- identify any treatable medical and psychiatric conditions which might be contributing to the memory impairment
- counsel patients and families about the illness
- refer promptly to other support services.

They utilise the skills of the geriatrician, psychiatrist of old age, clinical psychologist and clinical social worker and they aim to provide a multidisciplinary assessment for people aged 55 years and over with memory problems more than six months duration.
The three clinicians interview the patient separately and a

consensus opinion is formed. The **clinical psychologist** endeavours to determine the presence or absence of global cognitive impairment: this usually involves a face-to-face interview, followed by tests of verbal and visual memory, new verbal learning and visual constructional skills, mental speed, attention and orientation. The **geriatrician** identifies physical conditions that might be independently responsible for memory loss, pays particular attention to medication review and orders appropriate blood tests and additional investigations such as ECG, EEG and CT when clinically indicated. The psychiatrist performs a mental state examination to uncover disorders such as anxiety or depression contributing to the memory problem. He/she weighs the evidence for a diagnosis of dementia and normally uses the MMSE as a baseline test of performance which can be used again in follow-up. The **clinical social worker** joins in discussions about the patients, and offers comment about the degree of social, nursing and medical support that might be necessary. Thereafter, counselling is provided by a team member in the unit and later in the patients' homes.

At the Dundee Memory Clinic (McMurdo and Thompson, 1997) two-thirds of the patients referred have a diagnosis of probable dementia and the other third have affective disorders with remedial causes for forgetfulness or have been a subgroup of 'worried well'. It is obviously important in the latter group to remove the label of dementia from individuals who are not suffering from dementing illness.

The type of patient most suited for memory clinic referral are those who have had a short, atypical illness with memory and cognitive skill loss.

Patients who have well-established dementia with major behavioural problems, putting themselves or others at risk, are best referred to psychogeriatric services. Memory clinic staff support the concept of telling patients about their condition if they are still able to understand its significance. The diagnostic revelation provides an opportunity for the patient to be involved in future care preferences and helps family carers who are often relieved to learn that the patient's behaviour is the result of a real disease. It also gives family members an explanation for the often bizarre and incomprehensible behaviour demonstrated by their loved one.

5
The differential diagnosis

Age-associated memory impairment

Dementia is not part of normal ageing and has to be distinguished from benign senile forgetfulness, sometimes known as age-associated memory impairment (AAMI), where the name of an object or person may be forgotten, but associated details of the context can be remembered (Absher and Cummings, 1994). Its validity as a clinical entity has been questioned (Bayer and Woodhouse, 1993) on the grounds that it encompasses most early cases of dementia. Some American researchers believe diagnostic categories can be separated (Crook et al, 1986). Others doubt this (Blass, 1996), and there are no uncontroversial biological markers of AAMI at present.

The occasional memory lapse that comes with increasing age, particularly in the ability to encode and retrieve information, does not necessarily presage the catastrophic failure of mental facilities associated with dementia. Research at Manchester University Age and Cognitive Performance Research Unit has shown in a large prospective study of volunteers that the speed with which people can process information declines sharply with age, but memory skills alter relatively independently, usually with very small changes (Rossor, 1994). This work refutes the hypothesis that mental and other bodily functions decline rapidly just before death.

Ageing leads to deterioration in memory performance and older patients admit to worries that their inability to recall names may be the first part of a dementing process.

AAMI is the term used to describe the mild memory decline of old age, as opposed to the malignant changes that occur with a dementing process. Many believe AAMI to be non-progressive, and an identifiable condition with diagnostic criteria which does not appear to be a precursor of dementia (Hanninen et al, 1995). However, in this sub-group of people there will be some people with incipient Alzheimer's disease (Blass, 1996).

The majority of cases of dementia (over 50%) are caused by Alzheimer's disease. It is the major cause of dementia in elderly people. The second most common cause is multi-infarct dementia followed by

Lewy body type dementia (LBTD). A considerable number of people with dementia suffer from both Alzheimer's disease (AD) and multi-infarct dementia. It has become more important to try to identify the type of dementia present as new drug therapy appears to be more effective in LBTD than in ATD.

Differential diagnosis of types of dementia

The diagnosis of dementia is difficult, even for those skilled in dementia care, because dementia symptoms are diverse and non-specific (McLean, 1987). There are problems in distinguishing dementia from other treatable conditions, ie. stroke disease, acute confusion, depression and anxiety states.

The diagnosis is particularly difficult in the early stages when symptoms are not unlike the memory changes associated with ageing. There is no definitive test for dementia (Rossor, 1993; Sutcliffe, 1990) and accurate diagnosis depends on long-term assessments (O'Neill *et al*, 1982).

There is ample evidence to suggest that GPs are unaware of a significant number of patients with dementia (Iliffe, 1992; O'Connor *et al*, 1988). Misdiagnosis, where cognitive impairment is attributed erroneously to a functional psychiatric disorder, usually depression and overdiagnosis, where a non-dementing illness is diagnosed as dementia (Gordon, 1991), are not uncommon.

Differential diagnosis of differing types of dementia is important in order to exclude conditions which may be reversible with treatment if diagnosed early (see Figure 5.1). The three most common types of dementia are ATD, vascular dementia and LBTD.
The *Diagnostic and Statistical Manual of Mental Disorders* (DSM-IV) (American Psychiatric Association, 1994) sets out criteria for the diagnosis of various types of dementia. These have now been validated.

The differential diagnosis

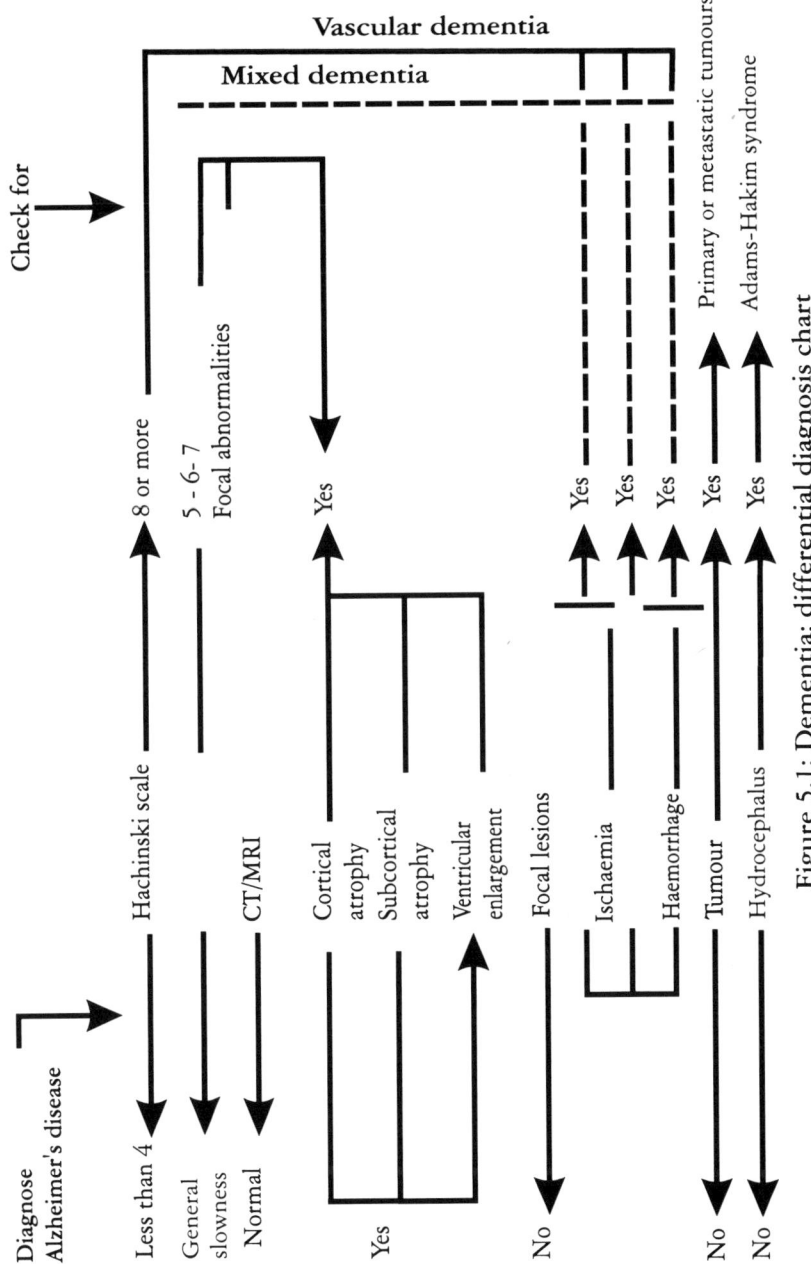

Figure 5.1: Dementia: differential diagnosis chart

Alzheimer's disease

DSM-IV criteria for diagnosis of Alzheimer's disease

These are considered in terms of mild, moderate and severe disturbance.

In mild ATD, work or social activities are significantly impaired but the patient can live independently without problems in personal hygiene and judgment is intact.

With patients with **moderate** ATD, independent living is hazardous in terms of personal care and some degree of supervision is necessary.

At a **severe** level of involvement, activities of daily living are so impaired that supervision is required all the time. Personal hygiene skills are lost and the patient may exhibit incoherence, aphasia and immobility.

All other specific causes of dementia should be excluded in clinical diagnostic terms. Confirmation of the diagnosis of AD requires:
- deficits in two or more areas of cognition, ie. perception, reasoning, intuition and the thinking processes
- progressive worsening of memory
- onset from 45 years of age
- steady decline in cognitive function and intellectual capacity
- absence of systemic disorder
- an alert individual showing no disturbance of consciousness.

The main elements are:
- decline in cognitive function
- abnormal score on memory testing
- neuropsychological abnormalities in two different cognitive areas such as memory and thinking
- absence of delirium.

Primary Alzheimer's disease can, however, present as delirium, delusions and depression as well as being untainted by such manifestations. These factors complicate diagnosis and have to be constantly remembered.

The differential diagnosis

Alzheimer's-type dementia:
- onset often insidious
- disease progresses over years
- course stable and then progresses
- alertness usually normal
- recent and sometimes remote memory can be impaired with perseveration relating to past events
- visual hallucinations occur in 30–40% of cases
- emotions are shallow, labile and apathetic
- orientation may be normal, but is more commonly impaired for time and place
- sleep can be disturbed with sundowning and nocturnal wandering
- sundowning may be a feature with late afternoon restlessness.

The ability to differentiate between types of dementia will become more important as new drugs become available for use in treatment. It is useful to remember that:

> *Alzheimer's disease* is gradual in onset, usually occurs in people over 45 and is progressive with global deterioration. It has been classified as early onset or late onset disease with the cut-off being arbitrarily set at 60–65 years of age (Rubinsztein, 1995). Mean age of diagnosis is 75 years (Jöst and Grossberg, 1995).

Multi-infarct dementia

Multi-infarct dementia (MID) has an onset from about the age of 55 onwards. In differentiation there is a marked early variable symptomatology and fluctuation in cognition with changes often occurring within the space of a day and from day to day.

MID can occur abruptly. There may be localising neurological signs and a possible past history of falls, intermittent confusion and speech difficulties, transient ischaemic attacks or cerebrovascular problems. Progression is often stepwise, with a step-by-step decline in skills and affect and intermittent personality change. Hypertension is common in these patients and if present there is usually evidence of other ischaemic heart disease. There may be a potential source of thromboembolism such as atrial fibrillation, vascular heart disease or carotid vessel disease. Differentiating features are the medical history, the abrupt onset of clinical features and the stepwise progression of the disease (see Chapter 2).

Lewy body-type dementia

In LBTD there are often florid visual and auditory hallucinations as well as delusions. The patient may also have a history of repeated unexplained falls or transient loss of consciousness and show mild evidence of Parkinson's disease (PD), such as rigidity, tremor, marked shuffling gait and poor tolerance of neuroleptic drugs (McKeith et al, 1994). Despite the fluctuating pattern the clinical features persist over a long period (weeks or months), unlike delirium which rarely persists as long. The illness progresses, often rapidly, to an end stage of severe dementia.

Other types of dementia

Vitamin B_{12} deficiency: This disorder is associated with anaemia and behavioural changes. Folic acid levels are often low and there may be sensory nerve changes in the legs and arms.

Hypothyroidism: This may cause a marked confusional state. It can also develop gradually if there is overtreatment of hyperthyroidism.

Parkinson's disease related dementia: This affects 10–20% of patients with PD. Parkinsonian features usually predate the onset of dementia. Apathy, poor concentration and indecision are dominant features. Parkinsonian features usually respond to dopaminergic drugs.

Progressive supranuclear palsy: This condition is similar to PD but the parkinsonian features do not respond to dopaminergic drugs.

Primary and secondary tumours: These may cause confusional states and may be identified by other localising symptoms. With frontal lobe tumours there can be disinhibited and irrational behaviour, mental apathy and indecision. Evidence of raised intracranial pressure may present late.

The differential diagnosis

When faced with difficult decisions regarding diagnosis it is useful to remember the **features of different types of dementia:**

1. Alzheimer's disease is gradual in onset, usually occurs in people over 45 years of age and is progressive with global deterioration. It predominates in those over 70 years of age.
2. MID may be of early onset, from the age of 55 years onwards, and often occurs suddenly with localising neurological signs such as transient ischaemic attacks. The history often reveals hypertension and cardiovascular problems and progression often shows a stepwise decline in skills and emotions and intermittent personality changes.
3. In LBTD there is usually some evidence of arterial vascular disease elsewhere and localising neurological signs with visual hallucinations.
4. Hypothyroidism is now relatively rare, but hyperthyroidism is not uncommon and over-treatment may lead to the development of pseudodementia.
5. Vitamin B_{12} deficiency is associated with anaemia and changes in behaviour can occur. Folic acid levels are often low and there may be sensory nerve changes in the legs and arms.
6. Primary and secondary tumours are not uncommon in the elderly.

> The path to a firm and accurate diagnosis of dementia is not always an easy one but a wide-reaching global approach to symptoms should lead to success.

Confusional states

At first presentation, dementia can be confused with delirium and chronic confusion. Confusional states are often reversible and it is important to recognise them so that appropriate treatment can be instituted. Unfortunately, in patients with dementia some symptoms are also features of acute delirium. Toxic confusional states complicate diagnosis but it is important to unearth alternative causes for dementia in the hope of improving mental and physical states.

> Approximately 10% of those who initially present with dementia will have a possibly reversible cause with the potential for cure with appropriate treatment.

Differentiating delirium and dementia

Usually in delirium:
1. Onset is acute.
2. Duration is usually short, over hours or days and is often only helpful in diagnosis in retrospect.
3. The course fluctuates, with lucid periods of consciousness, and is often worse at night.
4. Alertness is variable.
5. Orientation is often impaired in time, person and place.
6. Thoughts may be bizarre, paranoid and grandiose.
7. Perception may be disturbed with visual and auditory hallucinations.
8. Memory will show recent impairment.
9. Affect will be disturbed with other people, with the patient irritable, apprehensive and aggressive.
10. Sleep is likely to be disturbed with marked periods of nocturnal confusion.

Acute confusion

Acute confusion can result from:

1. Intoxication	Drug intoxication (including chronic intoxication
	Drug withdrawal (especially benzodiazepines)
	Alcohol intoxication/withdrawal
	Interactions of prescribed medicines

2. Infection	Urinary tract
	Respiratory tract
3. Water and electrolyte disturbance	Dehydration
	Hyponatremia
4. Hypoxia	Acute or chronic, eg. low cardiac output as a consequence of myocardial infarction or cardiac arrhythmias
5. Abnormal cerebral circulation	Transient ischaemic attack
	Stroke
6. Endocrine/metabolic disturbances	Hypo/hyperthyroidism
	Hypo/hyperglycaemia
	Hypo/hypercalcaemia
	Uraemia
7. Malnutrition	
8. Trauma	Subdural haematoma
	Subarachnoid haemorrhage
9. Intracerebral lesions	Tumour
	Normal pressure hydrocephalus

Depression and dementia

Depression is sometimes mistaken for dementia and vice versa (Burns and Hallewell, 1995). There are no confirmative diagnostic tests for either condition and diagnosis depends on history and observation. Both tend to be underdiagnosed in elderly people. To complicate matters further, depression frequently coexists with Alzheimer's disease the reported incidence being 57% (Lazarus et al, 1987; Liston, 1978).

Awareness of developing symptoms of dementia may precipitate patients into depressive illness. The term pseudodementia refers to cognitive impairment secondary to a primary depressive illness. Although the co-presentation of depression and dementia is not an infrequent occurrence, there is poor recognition that the depressive component is potentially treatable. In one recent study 86% of elderly patients with depression and dementia responded to antidepressive therapy and 80% of those in whom the depression lifted showed improvements in their Mini-Mental State Examination (MMSE) scores (Ancill, 1989).

However, many clinicians fail to recognise depression in demented individuals or have an ageist or nihilistic response to treatment (Katona and Katona, 1996). Conventional *Diagnostic and Statistical Manual of Mental Disorders* (American Psychiatric Association, 1994) (DSM-IV) criteria for a depressive diagnosis are of little value in recognising the condition in old people with dementia. Emphasis has to be given to behavioural changes exhibited by the patient. Ancill (1989) has suggested that the presence of two or three or more specific DSM-IV criteria for more than two weeks support a diagnosis of depression in a cognitively impaired patient.

Risk factors for depression in older people

Past history of depression
Positive family history of depression
Dementia
Myocardial infarction
Severe arthritis
Loneliness

The best way to increase the rate of detection is to have a high index of suspicion. Neither dementia nor depression is an inevitable sequela of old age. Many depressed old people present with somatic rather than psychological complaints, eg. tiredness, disturbed sleep, anorexia and weight loss. They may also display a high level of worry and personality changes resulting in care-seeking behaviour. Depressive thoughts such as guilt, reduced self-esteem, worthlessness, hopelessness and a preoccupation with death often mark the depressed patient who may also be suicidal. Some depressed people show abnormalities on cognitive testing, usually as a result of impaired concentration and attention, and occasionally present with impaired memory, but this usually has a more acute onset and a shorter history than dementia.

The differential diagnosis

Patients with dementia do not usually consistently complain of memory loss, and a failure to cooperate with cognitive testing suggests depression rather than dementia. The use of a depression assessment scale (Sheikh and Yesavage, 1986) (see Appendix 6) can often be of considerable value in this instance along with the use of a cognitive testing scale such as a memory test (see Appendix 6). The screening questionnaire recommended by the Royal College of General Practitioners is the Geriatric Depression Scale (GDS) (Appendix 6).

> Between 15 and 20% of people aged over 65 suffer from depressive order.
> Patients may present with the three Ds associated with Alzheimer's disease: dementia, delirium and depression.

Features of depression in the cognitively impaired:
1. Fitful sleep with many distressed awake periods
2. Loss of weight and poor appetite
3. Generalised fatigue and lethargy
4. Non-specific dysfunctional behaviour such as agitation, verbal and physical aggression
5. Diurnal variation in dysfunctional behaviour
6. Non-specific psychotic symptoms such as paranoia.

Other features distinguishing depression from dementia (Table 5.1):
1. Onset is often gradual
2. Illness may span weeks rather than months
3. Course — affect is usually more depressed in the morning and improves as the day goes on
4. Normal alertness
5. Normal orientation
6. Thoughts are often slowed and there is a sadness and hopelessness about the patient
7. Perception — 20% of depressed patients have mood-congruent auditory hallucinations
8. Emotions — sad, fearful, unresponsive and total flattening of affect.
9. Memory — recent memory is only occasionally impaired in depression, but remote memory is intact
10. Sleep — early morning wakening is common.

The summary in Table 5.1 can prove useful in differentiating a diagnosis of depression or dementia.

Table 5.1: Differentiating depression and dementia

	Depression	Dementia
History		
Onset	Dated from history	Vague
Progression	Can be rapid	Slowly progressive
Duration of symptoms	Short or long	Long
Family	May be aware of disabilities early on	Often unaware of disability until later
Symptomatology		
Memory loss	Patients complain of loss	Patients rarely complain of loss
Disability	Patients may emphasise disability	Patients hide disability
Time	Often worse in the morning Awaken in the early hours Difficulty in getting to sleep	Confusion worse in the evening Turns night into day
Investigations		
Computerised tomography	Scant evidence of atrophy	Cerebral atrophy and ventricular enlargement
Electroencephalogram	Usually normal	Pronounced slow activity
Single photon emission tomography	Blood flow patterns normal	Parieto-temporal and frontal abnormalities
Assessment scales		
BASDEC	High score	May be normal score
Hamilton depression	High score	May be normal score
AMT	Low score	High score
MMSE	Low score	High score
GDS	High score	May be normal

AMT   Abbreviated Mental Test Scale (Appendix 5)
BASDEC   Brief Assessment Schedule Depression Cards

The differential diagnosis

Hamilton D   Hamilton Depression Rating Scale
MMSE   Mini-Mental State Examination
GDS   Geriatric Depression Scale (Appendix 6)

If, after careful history-taking, there is still a diagnostic dilemma it is sometimes advisable to compare the symptoms of delirium, depression and dementia (Table 5.2).

Table 5.2: Clinical features of dementia, delirium and depression

	Dementia	Delirium	Depression
1. Onset	Insidious	Acute	Gradual
2. Duration	Months/years	Hours/days/weeks	Weeks or months
3. Course	Stable and progressive (unless MID — usually stepwise)	Fluctuates — worse at night Lucid periods	Usually worse in morning, and improves as day goes on
4. Alertness	Usually normal	Fluctuates	Normal
5. Orientation	May be normal — usually impaired for time and place	Always impaired — time, place, person	Usually normal
6. Memory	Recent and sometimes remote impaired memory	Recent impaired	Recent may be impaired Remote intact
7. Thoughts	Slowed Reduced interests Perseverate	Often paranoid and grandiose. Bizarre ideas, topics	Usually slowed. Preoccupied by sad and hopeless thoughts
8. Perception	Normal Hallucinations occur in 30–40% (often visual)	Visual and auditor hallucinations common	20% have mood-congruent auditory hallucinations
9. Emotions	Shallow, apathetic, labile, Irritable, careless	Irritable, agressive, fearful	Flat, unresponsive or sad and fearful. May be irritable
10. Sleep	Often disturbed. Nocturnal wandering common	Nocturnal confusion	Early morning wakening
11. Other features		Other physical disease may not be obvious	Past history of mood disorder

Further investigation may be required to separate out the diagnosis:
- *Computed tomography*: will demonstrate cerebral atrophy and ventricular enlargement in dementia whereas there will be scant evidence of atrophy in the depressed patient.
- Flow charts and comparison tables can sometimes help to resolve the diagnostic dilemmas that present when attempting to differentiate dementia due to cerebral pathology from other conditions.
- Some of the causes of confusional states will be identified after blood investigation which should include a full blood count, thyroid function, renal and liver function tests, vitamin B_{12} and folate levels, and serum calcium levels. The need for chest and skull X-rays may also become obvious on full medical examination.
- *Single photon emission computed tomography*: will show normal blood flow patterns in the depressed patient compared with temporal and frontal abnormalities in the dementing patient.
- A high index of suspicion for the presence of depression should be the norm. Where dysfunctional behaviour is the presenting problem, depression can be a major underlying cause when there is co-presentation of depression and dementia. Treatment of the depression will lead to an improvement in behaviour. The clinician also has to keep in mind that the presentation of early dementia is often precipitated by an additional treatable problem such as depression.
- In depression the *electroencephalogram* is usually normal, whereas in dementia there will be pronounced slow activity.
- *Hachinski ischaemic rating scale*: The use of the Haschinski ischaemic rating scale can assist in identifying the vascular-induced dementias. The Hachinski scoring device can also help to differentiate between vascular dementia and ATD. A total score of 4 or less is suggestive of ATD (Hachinski, 1974) (see Appendix 2). Vascular dementia is diagnosed when the patient scores 7 or higher. The Hachinski scale is widely used, despite poor inter-rater reliability, but it has practical value as part of a full assessment programme.
- *Depression rating scales*: may be useful in identifying depression.

Memory tests

There is no international concensus concerning the set of basic cognitive tests which should be used to assess dementia. Clinical rating and brief mental status scales are used to give a quick and global evaluation of dementia. GPs have been criticised for failing to carry out memory tests on initial assessment for dementia patients (Alzheimer's Disease Society, England 1995). Psychometric tests are valuable pointers towards diagnosis. They need not take long (Wilcock *et al*, 1994) and two tests that are widely used are the MMSE (Folstein *et al*, 1975) — Abbreviated Memory Test (AMT) (Hodkinson 1972).

The MMSE takes only 10 minutes to perform but can detect up to 90% of dementia and delirium cases (Anthony *et al*, 1982). These screening instruments are not full, definitive memory assessments, but can provide much valuable information about cognitive status. They are also of value when repeated at regular intervals, which is possible with annual geriatric assessment. They can easily be incorporated into geriatric assessment protocols. Community nurses who are accustomed to administering these scales can identify up to 96% of patients with moderate or severe dementia. However, they are slightly more likely than GPs to overdiagnose in this respect.

Nevertheless, the community nurse or geriatric health visitor can be a valuable asset in carrying out these preliminary tests. GPs and nurses are often reluctant to use assessment tools of this nature in practice, but they need not be time-consuming. No assessment of a patient with a possible dementing process should be completed without carrying out one of these tests.

People who complain of poor memory and memory- related problems have been shown to perform poorly on tests of memory and memory-related functions (Jonker *et al*, 1996). However, current evidence suggests that self-report of impaired memory alone is not useful to the clinician seeking to identify people with mild cognitive impairment (Wilson and Evans, 1996).

Further investigations for possible vascular dementias

> All patients with possible vascular dementia need careful assessment to detect any underlying causes and risk factors that might be remedial (Amar and Wilcock, 1996).

Selective investigation

Investigations should be tailored to the individual.
Ultrasonography will be required for patients with possible carotid artery stenosis.
Blood coagulation and *plasma viscosity* studies are indicated to identify hyperviscosity syndromes.
CT and MRI brain scans may identify specific treatable causes of dementia or frontal lobe tumour.
Ambulatory 24-hour blood pressure monitoring may identify hypertension which can cause cognitive impairment on its own (Amar and Wilcock, 1996).
Diabetes and hypercholesterolaemia can have a similar effect and should prompt blood screening to exclude these possibilities.
Blood investigations as detailed in Chapter 4 should be performed and should include:

- plasma viscosity and coagulation studies for antiphospholipid antibodies
- proteins C and S, antithrombin III and serum ascorbic acid assay (Gale et al, 1996).

Serum ascorbic acid assay may point to the need for dietary vitamin C supplementation or enhancement.
A search for vascular risk factors is important as vascular dementia is preventable. Controlling risk factors such as hyper- tension and diabetes and the use of antiplatelet drugs can improve cognitive function (Amar and Wilcock, 1996). Special attention should therefore be given to *examination of the cardiovascular system* as this is often a source of thromboembolism due to:

- atrial fibrillation
- heart failure
- valvular heart disease
- carotid stenosis

And should prompt:
- doppler ultrasonography of carotid arteries
- echocardiography — including 24-hour monitoring.

Neurological examination should also be undertaken, seeking evidence of:
- focal neurological deficit
- pyramidal tract signs
- dysarthria
- extrapyramidal signs.

Cognitive function in elderly people has been associated with death from ischaemic stroke. Those with greatest cognitive impairment have been found to have the lowest vitamin C serum levels. A high vitamin C intake may protect against cognitive impairment and cerebrovascular disease (Gale and Martyn, 1996).

There is an increased risk of vascular dementia in the presence of:
- stroke history (especially left-sided stroke)
- hypertension
- myocardial infarction history
- diabetes
- non-educational status
- cerebral atrophy
- cortical infarcts.

Korsakoff's syndrome

Korsakoff's syndrome (KS) is a chronic state characterised by loss of short-term memory induced by chronic alcoholism. Pathologically the hypothalamus sustains the most damage, whereas most other dementias are caused by damage to the cortex. KS is closely related to Wernicke's encephalopathy (WE) which is an acute-onset confusional state. Eighty-four per cent of those with WE develop KS (Victor *et al*, 1989). Both conditions are caused by a deficiency of Vitamin B_1. Technically, KS is not a true dementia since it does not have the usual degenerative and global features associated with other dementias.

Diagnosis: Typically there are three main features of WE — confusion, ataxia and ocular palsies — although they may not all be present. Symptoms can be confused with alcoholic withdrawal symptoms of ataxia, delirium and restlessness. KS cannot be accurately diagnosed until the patient has abstained from alcohol for four weeks.

Psychological features of KS: KS is characterised by memory loss, especially for events occurring after the onset of the condition, and retrograde amnesia. Memory loss is not always total and can improve with treatment. There is also an inability to acquire and store new information. Confabulation and lack of foresight with regard to memory loss are predominent features.

Blood investigations: Liver function tests and serum gamma glutamyl transpeptidase estimation.

Treatment: This is dependent upon prompt accurate diagnosis. WE is treated with intravenous or intramuscular injection of vitamin B_1. KS requires long-term vitamin B_1 dietary supple- mentation and abstinence from alcohol.

Down's syndrome and dementia

The mean life expectancy of people with Down's syndrome used to be very short but is now greater than 45 years and it is estimated that 20% of people with the syndrome are now in their fifth or sixth decade of life. These people have three rather than two copies of the chromosome 21. As the gene coding for amyloid precursor protein is localised on chromosome 21, this protein is therefore produced in excess. Amyloid is found to be deposited in the brains of people with Down's syndrome and in those with Alzheimer's disease, but knowledge of its causation and associations is still limited.

Characteristic neuropathological changes of dementia are found in the brains of people with Down's syndrome who are over 30 years of age at the time of death. Lai and Williams (1989) reported that 6% of 30-year-old people with the syndrome have dementia and that the figure rises to 75% in those over 55 years of age. If these patients show psychiatric deterioration in later life a diagnosis of dementia must be considered, but it is also important to exclude other causes such as hypothyroidism and depression in the differential diagnosis.

Parkinson's disease and dementia

PD and dementia can coexist. Follow-up studies on people with PD have shown that they have a more than threefold increased risk of developing dementia compared with controls. Among patients aged 50–54 years, the prevalence of dementia has been shown to be 13 times greater than in a similar age group of the general population (Breteler *et al*, 1995). This association of the two diseases should be kept in mind, as patients with both conditions will place even greater demands upon their carers.

Early onset dementia

Early onset dementia is now the preferred term for what was once called presenile dementia. The term describes a dementing process that starts before an arbitrary age of 65 years. However, this is an artificial distinction. Jorm and Korten (1988) suggest that seven per 1000 people aged 60–64 years may be affected by early onset dementia, with a prevalence of 34.6 per 100 000 in the 45–64 age group. Early onset dementia has been associated with an abnormal gene on chromosome 14 which leads to the mutated form of amyloid precursor protein, resulting in a higher production of amyloid.

GPs will only occasionally have to care for such individuals, but since early death in these patients is uncommon, they may have to care for them for a long time. A third die at home or in residential homes, so the family doctor will look after them for many years while they have been in community care. That care has been criticised. Only 18% of patients in one study felt that they had been given sufficient information at diagnosis concerning the progressive nature of the disease. Many were uninformed of support services and community care arrangements were often inadequate. The interval between symptom onset and firm diagnosis (mean 37.6 months) is longer for these patients than for older people with dementia (Jöst and Grossberg, 1995).

The social disruption caused by the onset of dementia at this early age is disproportionate to the numbers involved, and the NHS and support services are poorly organised to deal with this problem. Patients are too old for the preventive rehabilitative machinery in place for the young mentally ill, and too young for the services tailored for older people with dementia. They fall between two stools and the initial diagnosis of their condition is often delayed. Their needs are often inadequately met, being fitted into existing service provision by service providers picking and choosing between a range of services organised for other groups. Sometimes patient and carer have to struggle along alone because no service is identified as appropriate to their requirements. A flexible intervention programme is required to meet their special needs (see Appendix 4).

These cases of early-onset dementia present special problems in diagnosis, often because the doctor does not consider the possibility of dementia. The condition is misdiagnosed as depressive illness in 25% of cases (Newens *et al*, 1994). At initial contact with GPs, 48% of the patients were unaware that they had an ominous presenting problem. The GP's role in obtaining a confirmed diagnosis and co-ordinating support for patients and relatives is of paramount importance with this condition.

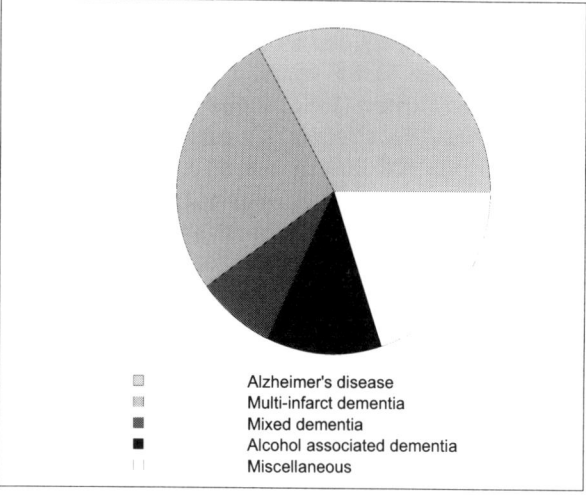

Figure 5.2: The subtypes of early onset dementia that presented to mental hospitals 1974–1988. From: Brooks and Whalley, 1992

6
The GP's role in management

Once differential diagnosis has been excluded and the diagnosis of dementia confirmed, assessment of the patient's and carers' needs have to be determined, and a management plan created. On average the patient is likely to live 7–9 years after the diagnosis of the dementia (Jost and Grossberg, 1995) and over much of this time will remain the responsibility of the family practitioner. The GP has a crucial role to play in liaison with the patient, family, carers, social work departments, the primary care team and hospital consultants and departments. Well placed to have a global overview of the patient's circumstances the GP can act as gatekeeper with a vital role in organising acute medical care, long-term institutionalisation when necessary and respite care admissions to diminish the load on the carer (see Figure 6.2). A unique knowledge of local services and awareness of the medical, functional and social status of the patient should permit family doctors to identify shortfalls and discrepancies in the care package and pressurise service personnel to fill the gaps (Smith, 1995). Sometimes, GPs alone have the status, as well as the trust of the patient, to negotiate acceptance of services for agreed admission to hospital or residential care when this has become essential and is being resisted.

A multidisciplinary avalanche of health and social workers can descend on the person with dementia on a one-off, intermittent or continuous intervention basis, in a well-intended care programme. This apparent overkill in service provision frequently disguises a marked limitation of effective support. Much of it will be sporadic, occurring within conventional social hours, when needs may not be predominant and support may be withdrawn without warning.

> The needs of the patient are not necessarily met by the apparent provision of high service input.

Case history:

> A patient of mine was being visited on 12 separate occasions by different agencies daily when her normal carer went on holiday. These interventions still did not prevent her lying for several hours on a stone floor in the cold when she fell and fractured her hip. The social service department had determined that it was cheaper to maintain her at home than in a residential home over this period. She might have been better cared for in a more secure situation than dependent upon the multiple irregular care visits which came her way.

There is evidence that service providers respond to those patients with demanding carers and many of the isolated, less vociferous and more socially deprived do not receive the service provision that their needs justify. The GP should be prepared to recognise shortfalls in service provision, endeavour to plug the gaps, and recognise the responsiblilty to maximise input of local and voluntary agency facilities to the patient's best advantage (see Figure 6.3).

Much of the continuing care of the patient can be delegated to nursing professionals, and local authority and social work departments (Figure 6.1). Although key workers from these disciplines may be involved it still falls upon the family practitioner to ensure that needs are being assessed on a regular basis and provision made for them wherever possible. The organisation of respite care and specialist service provision will fall to the GP and administrative staff. Needs have to be identified, problems recognised and regular global review instituted by the doctor.

This can be most easily done as part of the annual geriatric assessment programme (McIntosh, 1988) and by computer generation of review dates when health, functional and social status and provision of services can all be reviewed. This is facilitated by use of a standardised assessment procedure (see Appendix 4). Computerisation of data will make this an easier process, and review dates can generate a home visit by doctor or nurse. A holistic approach to the patient's, carers' and family's wellbeing should be embraced.

Figure 6.1: A multidisciplinary involvement in dementia care

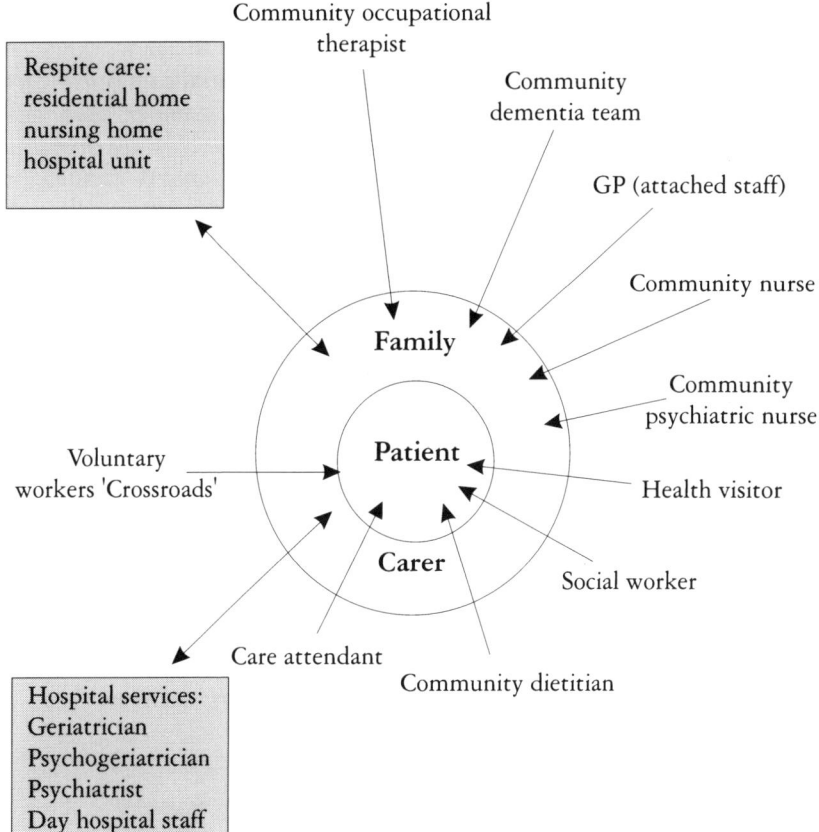

A structured approach to patient management will ensure good care and treatment of demented people and help to alleviate many of the problems experienced by those with the disease and their families.

Most of the day-to-day management of the patient will fall at the feet of the primary health-care team professional who becomes the key worker. He/she should be involved in the creation of the doctor's management plan. Objectives should be reasonable and based on pre-illness baselines and on assessment of new deficits and shortfalls in cognitive performance. Many of these patients have multiple problems and it is often necessary to prioritise them and deal with them one at a time. Ideally the patient should be informed of the plans, and the family should be involved in the planning stage.

There is a clear indication for review meetings of the primary health-care team, voluntary and family carers and social workers at least annually and ideally quarterly. This is an essential part of the care process, to ensure joint ownership of the management plan and maintain good communication between the many people involved in caring for a person with dementia. This involvement should be recognised as part of the GP's remit in patient care, although organisation can fall to the administrative staff. The GP, although usually not the key worker, can serve an important role in chairing or leading these meetings.

Meetings with relatives

An often forgotten feature is the need to educate relatives about future prospects regarding the disease and the patient's response to it. Pressures of time will limit GP commitment in this process, but it should be the GP's responsibility to ensure that this is done either personally or by a health professional colleague. There are times when it is particularly important to educate relatives:

1. When diagnosis is first confirmed.
2. When there is evidence of carer stress, eg. at times of anxiety, frustration, anger and depression.
3. When new behavioural problems arise.
4. When family circumstances change, and where shared care is threatened by the loss of a caring relative.
5. At a change to a different level of care, eg. inclusion of respite care, or more hospital involvement.

Guidelines for good practice

Guidelines for good practice from authoritative sources are proliferating, and the field of dementia has attracted attention. The Royal College of Physicians have produced guidelines on the management of acute confusional state. Evidence based clinical practice guidelines and interventions in the management and

Figure 6.2: A global approach to assessment — the patient's global environment

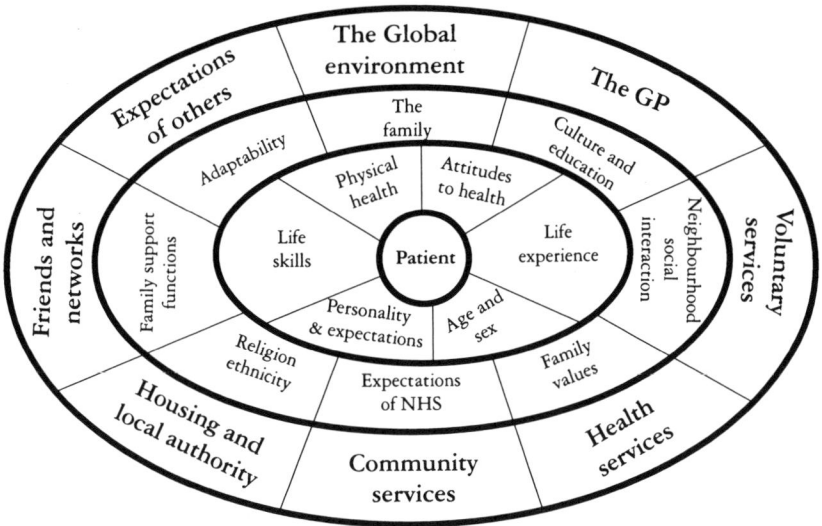

behaviour of psychological aspects of dementia have been produced for Scotland by the Scottish Intercollegiate Guidelines Network (SIGN) and the Department of Primary Care of the University of Newcastle has produced a guideline on the primary care management of dementia for the north of England. Many more guidelines particularly in relation to new drug management of dementia are due to appear. They can be a useful resource for busy GPs. They provide recommendations based on extensive reviews of the relevant literature and recommendations are usually explicitly linked to the evidence that supports them, with the degree of evidence published. The decision to adopt any particular recommendation lies with the individual practitioner. Guidelines are best regarded as useful reference tools, and attempts by colleagues with special interests and expertise in the field, to share an imperfect knowledge with clinicians, to ease the burden of management.

Acceptance of these recommendations outlined above commits the family doctor to:

1. Fully assess the physical, mental, behavioural and social problems of the person with dementia.
2. Assess the patient's remaining strengths and skills.
3. Identify and confirm the main diagnosis.
4. Identify any treatable, coexisting conditions.
5. Discuss the situation with an informed carer.
6. Identify the carer's specific problems and whether the carer's needs are being met.
7. Identify appropriate services required and liaise with service providers.
8. Review the needs of patient's care regularly — the GP's role is to monitor changing needs and identify new ones.
9. Consider early involvement of specialist services and specific cases.
10. Maintain a global overview of service provision from all the providers and be prepared to identify and plug the gaps.
11. Regularly visit the patient and carer at home or in the nursing home.
12. Record and analyse information obtained from the patient or carer on a regular basis, through care team meetings.

Several basic issues have to be kept in mind and reviewed from time to time, with input from discussions with other members of the care team:
- shortfalls in service provision will involve liaison with the social work department or local authority
- there may be conflicts of interest between the carer and the person with dementia, which may have to be identified and resolved, eg. consent of patient may have to be obtained to discourage further driving. Management of these issues should be discussed with the carer and key worker
- confidentiality concerns may have to be considered, eg. if the patient continues driving the GP has a duty to the community and may have to report this irregularity to the licensing authority
- considerations of power of attorney, curator bonis and

guardianship may have to be considered. The provisions of the Community Care Act 1990 will commit the social work department and long-term care will involve nursing homes, residential units and long-stay institutional care
- limitations of treatment and practice fund-holding considerations also have to be appraised.

The primary health care team's role in management

Responsibility can be delegated to attached local authority nurses, practice nurses, community nurses, community psychiatric nurses (CPNs) and health visitors (see Chapter 7).

The GP's role in the care team

The GP may only be practically involved in dealing with behavioural conditions requiring drug therapy, or, when the need arises, referral for a consultant opinion. The family doctor should, however, keep in mind that the prominent functional and social problems of these patients, which tend to dominate the management scene, can also coexist with medical and physiological decline, which may benefit from prompt appropriate therapeutic input (see Chapter 8). Close liaison with the team is important to ensure optimal quality of care.

Hearing loss and *visual difficulties* should be addressed and not neglected, and referrals as appropriate made to optician, ophthalmologist or audiometric specialist. These patients suffer from the same simple *chiropody* problems as their non-affected peers, and their mobility can be much improved by referral for appropriate chiropody care. Every endeavour should be made to keep them as physically healthy as any other ageing individual on the practice list. *Incontinence* in dementing patients merits the same investigations and efforts to ameliorate it as for any geriatric patient (see Chapter 9). Prompt treatment of urinary problems can make life easier for both patient and carer.

One frequently overlooked problem is the possibility of *malnutrition* in people with dementia. Berlinger and Potter (1991) has shown that in community-living patients there is an association between dementia and low body mass index. Other studies have shown that up to 50% of people with Alzheimer-type dementia (ATD) or multi-infarct dementia (MID) are either protein or calorie malnourished (Bucht and Sandman, 1990). Patients with ATD may require a higher energy intake than cognitively normal, elderly people (Renvall *et al*, 1993).

Investigation of food intake, possible malabsorption and the disease process have not determined reasons for such malnutrition. The SSRI drug fluoxetine induces anorexia in depressed patients (Kelsey, 1995). Nutritional intervention can improve cognitive behaviour possibly by reduction of episodes of hypoglycaemia. The GP should perhaps therefore consider the possibility of malnutrition especially in people with ATD and living alone, and enlisting the help of the community dietician (Archibald, 1994).

The relation between cognitive function and risk of death from stroke suggests cerebro vascular disease is an important cause of declining cognition. Cognitive performance in the elderly has been found to be poorest in those with lowest vitamin C status. A high vitamin C intake, supplied by two oranges per day, may protect against cerebro vascular disease and cognitive decline. A diet with high vitamin C content may be a useful recommendation for patients in the earliest stages of dementia (Gale, 1996).

Figure 6.3: Role of various health professionals and other supporting professionals and agencies in community care.
Source: Alzheimer's disease society (1995) *Dementia in the Community: Management Strategies for General Practice*, Alzheimer's Disease Society, London

Service Provider	FHSA	HA	SS	LA	VA	DSS	IR	PS
Screening								
Health promotion		•						
Memory clinic		•						
Assessment & treatment (medical and social)								
Consultant domiciliary visit	•	•						
Day hospital		•						
Old age psychiatry		•						
Neurologist								
In-patient and psychogeriatric services		•						
Community dementia teams		•	•					
Social worker			•					

The GP's role in management

Service Provider	FHSA	HA	SS	LA	VA	DSS	IR	PS
Respite care								
Day hospital		•						
Health visitor and district nurse		•						
Occupational therapist		•						
Physiotherapist		•						
Chiropodist		•						
Incontinence nurse		•						
Dementia therapies								
Reality orientation		•						
Cognitive stimulation		•						
Validation therapy		•						
Drug therapies		•						
Information and counselling								
Written information		•	•		•			
Support groups					•			
Community psychiatric nurse		•						
Health visitor and district nurse								
GP and practice nurse	•							
Hospital (including day hospital)		•						
Community support								
Meals on wheels			•		•			
Bathing/dressing (nursing)		•	•		•			•
Home help/care assistant			•		•			•
Transport			•	•	•			
Day care		•	•	•	•			
Holiday admissions		•	•	•	•			
Sitter services			•	•	•			
Family break schemes			•		•			
Financial help								
Attendance allowance/disability								
Living allowance care component						•		
Long-term residential care								
Part III homes			•					
Warden supervised accommodation					•			•
Residential homes			•		•			•
Nursing homes		•			•			•
Long-stay wards (including psychiatric and geriatric hospitals)		•						

FHSA	Family health services association
HA	Health authority
SS	Social services
LA	Local authority
VA	Voluntary agency
DSS	Department of Social Security
IR	Inland revenue
PS	Private supplier

The GP has a central role as family practitioner and advocate for the patient's needs, other supporting professionals and agencies.

Observations of people early in the course of dementia reveal considerable awareness and insight. The **'medical model'** approach to treatment should always involve social and psychological aspects of management (Briggs, 1993). Dementia is an 'existential plight' of person, not simply a problem to be investigated and managed through technical skill (Kitwood, 1988).

With many professionals involved (Figure 6.4), it is important that responsibilities are clearly defined, and that pressure is put upon the professionals to meet their commitments in what should be interlocking services devoid of gaps. Equally it is important that professional care-givers do not offer services and responses which cannot be provided, as this merely causes frustration and psychological disturbance in patients and carers. There will inevitably be overlapping of professional roles. The dangers arise when professionals assume that others are filling the gaps and no-one provides a needed service. This is a classic area for collusion between members of the workforce. All too frequently there is a failure in communication and none of the workers are aware of what the others are doing or, more importantly, are unaware of what is not being done. The GP is well placed to define the responsibilities of each of the professionals involved and to ensure that these are being met, and that support is seamless — an ideal that is rarely achieved.

Nursing home care

While GPs may have only a few patients with dementia living in the community, the majority will have responsibilities to patients in the many nursing homes which have proliferated in recent years. Perhaps half of these patients will have some degree of dementia. The quality of care for these patients is variable and has been questioned (McIntosh, 1996). Although their physical needs are generally attended to, those with mental disabilities often receive less than optimal therapeutic care. All too frequently, patients with dementia are herded into common rooms and left in front of the television set for many hours every day.

They are also at risk from oversedation and overprescribing of neuroleptics (McGrath and Jackson, 1996). GPs are under pressure from nurses and relatives to contain challenging behaviour by the use of medication and all too frequently such medication is repeated without being reviewed. The term 'warehousing' has been coined for these patients. The long-term state institution has been changed for a poorly controlled, privately run institution where patients are fed and watered, kept clean and dry, and then left to their own resources. The state and society have apparently met their obligations but these are far from ideal for the individual patient who lacks mental and sensory stimulation.

In the USA the majority of nursing home patients exhibit dementia, behavioural disturbance, psychosis or depression but very few receive appropriate mental health care; consequently such homes now serve as *de facto* mental institutions for older people (Rovner, 1996). A similar situation is developing in Britain, as demonstrated by the high and probably inappropriate prescription of neuroleptics in nursing homes. GPs, who are often unwillingly enlisted into caring for these patients, feel poorly trained and have little time to meet demands. Patients often do not get the attention they might receive if still living in the community. The patients merit the same attention to their physical and psychological status and social wellbeing as those living at home in the care of relatives who can ensure that appropriate medical and social attention is forthcoming. Many patients in nursing homes are bereft of visitors, become isolated from the community and depend upon professional carers to meet their needs. However, these are not always addressed.

Urinary tract infections are common in nursing home residents and are a cause of confusion in the old. They are often missed and urine testing should always be considered. Poor nutrition may result in **anaemia** which should be sought. Patients admitted with other conditions such as alcoholism and parkinsonism may develop dementia and this should be investigated and verified just as with any other patient on the practice list. **Depression** is a concomitant condition of dementia and its presence should be considered. The behaviour of many of these patients may be improved and they become more actively motivated and produce less challenging behaviour if the depression is treated. *Drug medication* should be kept to the minimum dose and not routinely prescribed without regular review.

If patients are kept physically fit, their mental capabilities will be optimised. Activity programmes will stimulate and improve patients' behaviour, but staff attitudes may need to be addressed and changed to encourage their implementation. Vitamin supplementation may improve mental performance in some patients. Once placed in the nursing or residential home situation these patients should be assessed. Many miss out on the annual geriatric surveillance, which theoretically would come their way if living in the community, and there is a tendency for them to be maintained on medication they were taking on arrival, which may become unnecessary once they are settled in the new care situation. Vulnerable individuals are at a considerable risk of exposure to exploitation and possible abuse factors (Ford and Heath, 1995) and attending doctors should keep this in mind. The care of community-living people with dementia is rightly criticised, but the care of those living in residential and nursing home also leaves much to be desired. Caring GPs can do much to improve the lot of such people, promote a change in attitude in professional carers and reduce the demands on primary carers.

Bureaucratic rules can exert a depersonalising effect and create dependency and 'learned helplessness' (Maier and Seligman, 1976). Powerlessness in the patient can lead to apathy, depression and behavioural disturbance in patients with cognitive disability. Paternalistic and defensive reactions by staff 'in the interests of safety' can bring restrictions in liberty, eg. the restraining chair, or drug-induced constraint, and are likely to occur when the patient's ability to cooperate and exercise personal competency is reduced. An individualised management plan and an 'active view' of nursing home care should be encouraged (Philips, 1992). This process can be expedited by the use of Dementia Care Mapping, a tool devised to measure the quality of the demented individual's experience (Kitwood, 1993).

GPs have a unique opportunity to encourage improved management of these patients, orchestrated towards a more active therapeutic programme. Activity programmes that have been developed specifically for use with people with dementia are available; such programmes promote exercise, sensory stimulation, reminiscence,

The GP's role in management

socialisation and self-esteem (Ritter, 1991). A visit to a vibrant, activity-rich nursing home unit attests to the presence of happier, more interactive patients. Activity programmes reduce the prevalence of behaviour disorders and the use of antipsychotic drugs (Rovner, 1996). Attending doctors can encourage nurses and management staff to provide this calibre of care for patients with dementia. An enhanced programme of therapeutic activity can reduce not only the demands made by nursing staff but also the considerable GP workload generated by nursing and residential home patients.

7
Roles of the care team

GPs' perceptions of the role of different members of the extended primary health care team and their importance vary (see Figure 7.2). Perceptions on principal role players also differ with a quarter of GPs believing that they have a principal role in the management of people with dementia (McIntosh et al, 1997).

Nursing attachment

The availability of health professionals varies markedly from area to area. Most GPs have practice nurses attending to the physical needs of elderly people in the community. They are well placed to deal with the supervision of medication, incontinence problems and organisation of service provision. Professional extensions of the nursing role, however, mean that they can also take a much more active part in caring for demented people in the community.

With appropriate instruction, they can assess communication difficulties, functional deficits and carer needs and be involved in global health management plans. In many practices, nurses are already responsible for annual geriatric assessment, which provides an ideal opportunity for them to be delegated specific responsibilities in terms of assessing patients with cognitive losses of a dementing nature. The traditional nurse's role involves:

1. Maintaining the patient's independence at a maximal level of individual ability.

2. Providing support for patients and relatives.

3. Liaison with other care team members.

Good nursing care of people with dementia extends this commitment. Nurse colleagues, with the support of GPs, should be taking a holistic and person-centred approach to the care of people with dementia, helping them to maintain the highest possible quality of life. The traditional biomedical model provides a rather passive and palliative role for a nurse. A much wider approach is required to deal with the multiplicity of cognitive, emotional and social problems associated with the dementing process (Watkins, 1988). Nurses should be encouraged to accept the confused behaviour of people with dementia as an understandable reaction of that person to the stresses of powerlessness, loss of personal control and social isolation which affect them.

A proliferation of techniques, such as reality orientation, reminiscence, validation, expressive therapy and life reviews (Janssen, 1988), have been embraced by nurses working enthusiastically in this field in the last few years. These techniques provide sensory stimulation to affected individuals and help them to maintain social skills — an endeavour to improve and maintain remaining cognitive abilities. They should be able to provide a flexible care service, based on a global view of the circumstances relating to the family but focused on the individual and used in combination with systematic assessment and a problem-solving approach to needs. Currently the nurse's role in giving information to carers and promoting carers' health with counselling and support is still underdeveloped. Nurses' input can be vital in a household where there is a demented patient. Nurses should be encouraged to develop positive and optimistic views with regard to the dementia and the capacity of people suffering from it and be committed to helping cognitively impaired patients live at ease with their impairment.

There has to be a shift from purely physical care to psychotherapeutic care, a bridge that some caring, conscientious nurses find difficult to cross. They need to acknowledge that their contribution to this kind of care extends beyond professional physical actions and includes their own behaviour, emotions and responses. They should endeavour to understand the patient's experience and comprehension of what has happened to him/her.

There has been a tendency for nurses to regard their care priority as a physical one rather than a psychosocial interaction with restorative activities (Brook *et al*, 1975). There is some evidence (Armstrong-Esther and Brown, 1986) that there are low levels of nurse/patient communication in this field, with nurses interacting significantly less often with confused patients than with lucid ones. Nurses may have to be encouraged to respond in the same way to confused and demented patients as they do to those with physical problems.

The Royal College of Nursing has published *Guidelines for Assessing Mental Health Needs in Old Age* (RCN, 1994). These aim to provide nurses with a framework for identifying and assessing mental ill health and dementia in particular. They emphasise a global approach, encompassing mood, cognition, behaviour, and social and biographical factors. The principles include selection of the right tools for the job, where and when to make an assessment, the development of interpersonal skills and relationships with patient and carer, and identification of the individual's needs, strengths and assets for an individualised nursing intervention plan.

The RCN clearly identifies the role of the nurse in assessing mental as well as physical needs and recommends that nurses create a home environment that promotes independence and aims to overcome mobility and cognitive impairment. The College encourages screening for dementia and medication surveillance and review (RCN, 1993).

The nurse can make use of several assessment tools:

Barthel Activities of Daily Living Index (ADL): This is the most commonly used ADL index. It covers ten basic aspects of daily activity and living and has proven reliability and validity. It is simple, quick and easy to use (Mahoney and Barthel, 1965) (see Appendix 3).

Memory test: Mini-Mental State Examination (MMSE) or Abbreviated Mental Test (AMT) (see Appendices 1 and 5).

Geriatric Depression Scale (Sheikh, 1986): A valid and reliable brief rating scale that is useful for screening for depressive symptoms as well as monitoring change. It can be completed in five minutes by an interviewer (see Appendix 6).

Elderly Assessment Profile and Checklist : Assessment can be mainly completed by the nurse. The doctor is responsible for the clinical section (see Appendix 4) (McIntosh, 1990).

Hachinski Ischaemic Score: See Appendix 2.

With GP support and encouragement, the attending nurse should develop a care plan for that particular patient, built on a needs assessment, based on a complete picture of patient function, family and social networks, social and economic situation. Nursing intervention should focus on strategies for dealing with the common problems such as verbal and non-verbal communication, physical functioning, perceptual and motor difficulties, memory loss and social isolation. Several care models are utilised in dementia management but two in particular are:
- patient orientated

- carer orientated.

Both of these models are based on a problem-solving approach. Nurses rapidly assess patients' nursing requirements using an ADL model. It is more difficult to identify priority needs for the care-giver and it may be useful to use an approach based on the dementia stress management model (see Figure 7.1).

Figure 7.1: Dementia stress management model for patient behavioural problems

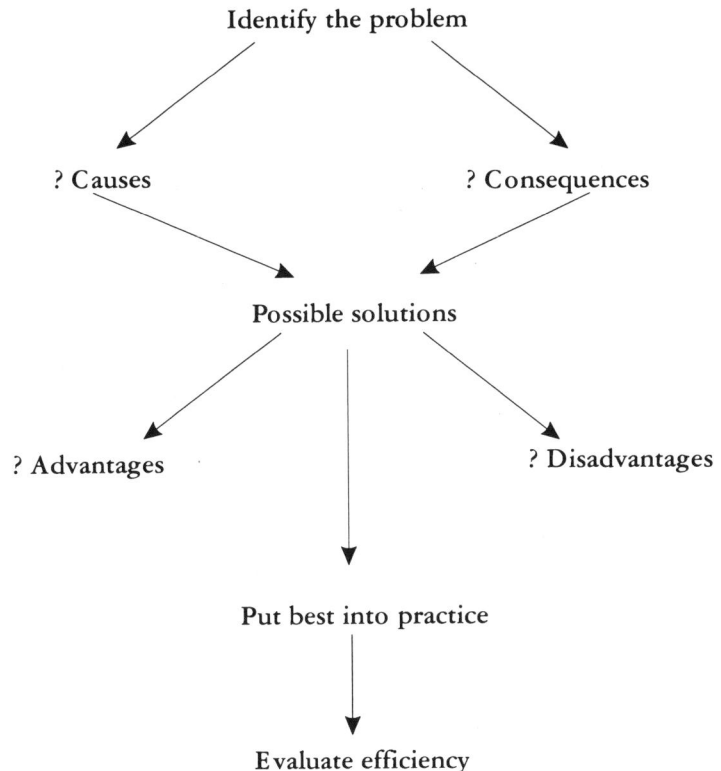

Traditional nursing duties have concentrated on physical care with priority given to alleviating obvious risks factors, mobilising retained skills and encouraging function in ADL. Emphasis has been placed on hygiene, eating and drinking skills, urinary and faecal control and problem behaviour.

A more holistic approach embraces:
- efforts to enhance communication
- appreciation of perceptual problems
- stress assessment in patient and carer
- emotional support to patient and carer
- making allowance for expressions of sexuality
- encouraging social interaction
- optimising the use of retained skills.

Nursing care should aim to encourage and support the patient's personal state of 'relative wellbeing' (Kitwood and Bredin, 1992).

Figure 7.2: Members of the primary care team perceived as the most useful by GPs

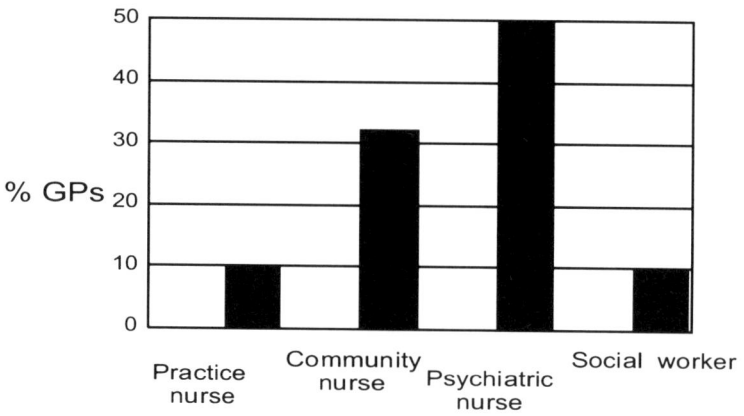

Practice nurses

Many GP-employed practice nurses are already involved in annual geriatric surveillance programmes, either opportunistically or by routine visits of the elderly. Their role can easily be extended to include screening for dementia and they have the ability to undertake home visits, provide physical nursing care and monitor the support required by the dementia patient and home carer (Alzheimer's Disease Society, 1995). As core members of the primary health care team, they are believed to have a special role to play in identifying people with early symptoms of dementia (Keady, 1996).

Nurse practitioners

Nurse practitioners have arrived on the general practice scene. Their focus is on health rather than disease (Stilwell, 1982), with the emphasis on holistic care. They can take full responsibility for their professional practice (Bowling, 1993). Their attention is given to areas where they can perform as well as or better than the doctor. Their patient assessment can incorporate physical examination and diagnosis to allow differentiation between normal and abnormal findings. This status is acknowledged by the Government (NHSME, 1993).

In this capacity, if trained, nurse practitioners are ideally placed to screen for dementia and to fulfil much of the comprehensive assessment and management of people with dementia and their carers.

Health link workers

Some practices, especially fundholders, are employing link workers, who are often partly trained health workers, for geriatric annual surveillance and screening purposes. My own practice has for many years used a two-year trained nurse to carry out this work in association with a health visitor. They carry out geriatric home visiting, complete geriatric assessment profiles and perform memory tests. They develop skills and expertise of value in screening for dementia, routine assessment of people with dementia, and assessing needs of patients and carers (McIntosh, 1990).

The health visitor

Health visitors are well placed to identify new cases of dementia and assist in diagnosis. However, many health visitors see their main job in terms of paediatric care, and most have limited training in psychiatry or geriatric medicine. In some areas, however, they are active in annual geriatric assessment and can easily extend their commitment, by conducting memory tests, to identify new cases of dementia.

Community occupational therapists (OTs)

OTs are now working more with people with dementia in the community and often provide the access route to additional functional aids. They are active in assessing ADL as well as instituting recreational activities. Not all have had the training, however, to enable them to assess patients' mental state, as well as physical state, to determine whether the aids provided will be effective. Some now practise the techniques of reality orientation, validation, reminiscence, resolution therapies and life review with their patients in the community. Many of these techniques can be taught by the nurse or OT to the immediate carer, and are often very effective in enhancing the patient's quality of life.

Community dementia teams

Community dementia teams operate in some areas. They comprise a group of statutory and voluntary professionals who work in association with the community memory clinic or psychogeriatric unit. They may be directly accessible to the GP. Team members will visit and arrange support and services and report back to the GP.

Community mental health teams (elderly)

These are usually geriatric or psychogeriatric consultant-led. They usually include community psychiatric nurses (CPNs), psycho- logists and social workers. GPs are often unaware of their existence and there is an obvious case for GPs and the team to establish a working relationship for the benefit of patients.

Community dietician

Help may be required for the malnutrition associated with dementia. This is a frequently overlooked problem and simple dietary measures may often improve the patient's quality of life.

Social workers

Social workers are often key personnel in determining entry to residential and nursing home care within the NHS. They are responsible for longer-term placement assessment, which is often carried out by a geriatrician on their behalf. They are currently struggling with the changes and responsibilities thrust on them by the Community Care Act, 1990 and some lack the expertise and skills to cope with a much changed situation. A diploma in geriatric care is being developed to allow social workers to educate themselves in this field. Long delays are not uncommon between referral, assessment and admission to long-stay units. The GP should consider early referral so that when the time of need does arise the social work department has at least made contact with the patient and has a patient profile on record. This may bring a quicker response to urgent requests for admission to long-term care. Social worker care managers now have a clearly defined role in the management of the elderly people with dementia and assessing the needs of family carers. In a study of social workers different perceptions of their social work role were revealed.

Perceived roles reported by social workers (MacMichael, 1995)

	%
Problem solver	57
Adviser on welfare rights	43
Mobiliser of resources	71
Diagnostician and planner	57
Agent of social control	71
Coordinater of services	71
Advocate and mediator	57

There has traditionally been conflict between family doctors and social work professionals, which might have been resolved if social workers had been attached to primary health care teams. The social worker's role and outlook have tended to be viewed with suspicion by GPs, an understandable view when the former have problems in perception of their own role — which, in the case of the elderly person in the community, has now been much more clearly defined. Where conflict in care objectives and managements do arise, the GP could usefully refer to the Dementia Services Development Centre (DSDC) book, *Peacemaking between tribes* (McMichael *et al*, 1995) for tips to ensure harmonious working relationships. Practices with attached social workers invariably develop a good professional association of benefit to colleagues and patients.

The local authority

Through its social service department the local authority is responsible for the provision of *home helps* or *care attendants*. These paid carers often play a crucial role in supporting people with a dementing process. They should be involved in the management decision process and can be usefully encouraged to see themselves as an extension of the health care team. Committed care attendant support is often all that stands between the person with dementia remaining at home or becoming institutionalised.

Social work department (SWD) services

SWD services vary markedly between authorities and across the country and it behoves the GP to be aware of what is available locally. The majority offer home, day and respite care with varying short- and long-term residential provision. More than a third of the residents in many local authority residential homes have a measure of dementia. SWD responsibilities now encompass the purchase of individualised care packages for elderly people in need. There is a widely recognised need for closer collaboration between GPs and the social services.

The GP's role in the multidisciplinary team

1. Provision of information about diagnosis and prognosis (Davies, 1988; Gilleard, 1984; Willcock, 1993).
2. Assessment of the carer's coping skills.
3. Provision of information about the support services and benefits (Gilleard and Willcock, 1993; Rossor, 1993).
4. Provision of emotional support for carers (Brodaty, 1988).
5. Gatekeeping in access and coordination of different support services.
6. Providing a global overview of events affecting patient and carer (Downs, 1994).

To perform these roles adequately the GP must be knowledgeable about access to the various services and the non-voluntary services available in the area. He/she should recognise the need to liaise between different services and help fill the care gaps. Informal carers, usually family members, are crucial to the success of community care of these patients and should be recognised by GPs as partners in the process of caring. It is important that doctors are committed to good communication between patient, family and carer in terms that carers can understand. Ensuring that supportive networks are in place, enabling the people involved to talk with each other — and with those who are responsible for service provision — may be the most important improvement to be made in the short-term.

Key components of community care

(Source: Department of Health (1989) *Caring for People. Community Care in the Next Decade and Beyond*. Cmd 849. HMSO, London.)

1. Services that respond flexibly and sensitively to the needs of individuals and their carers.
2. Services that allow a range of options for consumers.
3. Services that intervene no more than is necessary to foster independence.
4. Services that concentrate on those with the greatest needs.

Key objectives for service delivery:

- to promote the development of domiciliary, day and respite services
- to ensure that service providers made practical support for carers a high priority
- to make proper assessment of need and good case management the cornerstone of high quality care
- to promote the development of a flourishing independent sector alongside good quality public service
- to clarify the responsibilities of agencies.

Services provided by the local authority (DSDC, 1995b):

- *home care service* using either a general or specially trained

home care attendant
- *day care* in local authority residence or specialist unit
- *respite care* in residential homes, in the domiciliary situation
- *residential long-term provision*
- *relative support groups*
- *multidisciplinary patient reviews*
- *community mental health teams* — a key focus for the provision of services for older people with dementia. Some have community dementia teams
- *carer support* — time-limited emergency continuous care in the patient's home, eg. when the carer is unwell and hospitalised
- *drop-in centres* for people with dementia and carers
- *mobile emergency care schemes* — cruising road patrols which respond to triggering of passive alarms by people with dementia (McWhirter, 1987)
- *training for professional carers*
- *special provisions* for people with learning difficulties who have dementia, and for people under 65 years who have had early-onset dementia. This group is poorly catered for by the majority of local authorities (Marshall, 1994).

In-home respite care is provided by very few local authorities although this service appears to be the most sought after by carers (Downs, 1994).

In some areas, funding for the care of such individuals is based on a medical diagnosis of mild, moderate or severe dementia. This often results in people with mild dementia receiving less financial and social support than those with severe dementia, although their practical needs may not be very different. Someone with severe dementia, well supported by different networks, may need less support than someone with mild dementia living alone in squalid conditions. Staging the disease and thereafter labelling the patient in a similar fashion has its drawbacks, although the GP may be more comfortable with this traditional medical model.

Workers from other disciplines have criticised the traditional medical approach to dementia care, seeing it as a technical response. Kitwood (1993) likens it to the way that an AA breakdown mechanic deals with the car that will not start. The mechanical failure is remedied in some way to have the engine restart, but the defect has not been cured. Kitwood feels that the traditional approach can affect those suffering from dementia, for instance, by obstructing access to health and social care.

Good dementia care management should involve a willingness to embrace other care models. Kitwood (1988) would like dementia to be seen in much more personal terms from a broadened view. He has produced an equation:

Senile dementia = neurological impairment + personality + biography + health state + social psychology

and has further developed this approach. He maintains that much of the social psychology element is of a malignant variety which actually has a bearing on the level of neurological impairment of function in the affected individual. Traditional models tend to focus on events that have already happened, or on pathological changes, and are usually difficult to influence. Kitwood stresses the need to consider the effects of the responses from carers and others on the affected individual. Inappropriate responses can affect the individual and add to his/her impairment. The patient's behavioural disturbance may be related to the context of their social interactions and the responses and behaviour of others.

Generally, management will need to embrace 'problems' best dealt with one at a time. Ideally the patient, if capable of understanding, should be told of any plans that are drawn up and the family should be involved. The team meeting will define who is responsible for the management of the different problems. This is a problem-oriented approach with continuing day-to-day management often falling to the nurse or carer.

The Alzheimer's Disease Society (1995) has produced a management guide for dementia care, written specifically for the GP and endorsed by the Royal College of General Practitioners. This guide, together with its associated publications *A Practice Guide for Community Nursing* (Archibald et al, 1995) and *Dementia: A Practice Guide for Social Work Staff* (Burton et al, 1997) merit a place in every general practice library. Developed from a training guide (McLennan et al, 1993) for GP trainers and registrars, these publications are succinct, readable and have proved popular, up-to-date training aids.

8
Drug management of dementias and behaviour problems

Our ability to retard or improve cognitive impairment in Alzheimer's disease (AD) has advanced significantly in recent years. Possibilities for the therapeutic management of AD improved with the production of tetrahydroaminoacridine (tacrine). New generations of products are arriving on the scene that may be more effective and have fewer side-effects than tacrine. Several different pharmacological approaches have taken place in terms of therapy for Alzheimer-type dementia (ATD). These involve either neurotransmitters, neurotrophics or neurotrophic support strategies or are directed against specific disease mechanisms. Pharmacological treatment is mostly focused on improvement in memory and cognitive functions (Gottfries, 1994).

The marked depletion of the neurotransmitter acetylcholine in the cerebral cortex is the most common chemical abnormality in ATD. By the time of diagnosis, cortical acetylcholine synthesis is reduced to almost half in most patients, and by the time of death it may be down to one third. Changes in the cholinergic system have been shown to correlate well with a degree of cognitive impairment in ATD. This has encouraged the use of anticholinesterases, which retard the destruction of intrinsically produced acetylcholine and enhance cerebral cholinergic neurotransmission. Choline esterase inhibitors are a specific treatment for AD, rather than dementia in general.

Neurotransmitter-related drugs have also been used in an attempt to improve some of the behavioural and other non-cognitive symptoms of ATD. Certain neuronal systems are affected in ATD which are protected by neurotrophic proteins, such as nerve growth factor. The use of such proteins may provide the basis for halting, or at least retarding, the neuronal degeneration that is characteristic of AD.

Amyloid production and the production and processing of amyloid precursor protein (APP) have also excited biochemists. Drugs that alter the processing of APP may prove to be of therapeutic value. It seems likely that within the next few years, drugs will be marketed that will either retard or halt the progression of cognitive decline.

Lewy body-type dementia patients produce even less

acetylcholine than those with AD (Edwardson, 1994). There is some evidence that patients with this type of disease respond to drugs such as tacrine. With the advent of possible drug treatments for the underlying cognitive impairment it is becoming increasingly important to assess patients with this in mind. Wilcock *et al* (1994) consider that all potential patients should be screened, as at least some of those found suitable for treatment are likely to benefit from new drug therapy approaches.

Drug research approaches to ATD

Neurotransmitter related strategies

The most characteristic neurotransmitter abnormality in the brains of patients with ATD is a substantial deficit in presynaptic cholinergic neurones. This is reflected in a loss of subcortical cholinergic neurones, innervating the neocortex and hippocampus. Several acetylcholine esterase inhibitors are currently in advanced stages of development. These drugs are from different chemical classes: organophosphorous compounds, eg. metrifonate; carbamates, eg. physostigmine; Exelon; and benzylpiperidines.

The likely effect of these drugs is to increase the activation of post synaptic neurones with acetyl choline receptors, particularly glutamatergic pyramidal neurones. In ATD pathology, these latter cells are considered to be either lost or hypoactive, or the site of mismetabolism of amyloid precursor protein (APP) leading to the deposition of beta-amyloid protein.

Prevention of amyloid plaque formation

In familial ATD a defect in chromosome 21 will result in a pathological cleavage of the pre-amyloid protein. The formation of amyloid is considered the main pathological factor in ATD. The pharmaceutical industry is researching drugs that are capable of antagonising the deposition of the precursor protein, or delaying the maturation of beta-amyloid protein.

Non-specific anti-inflammatory drugs (NSAIDs)

In one study, involving a six year prospective survey of 7,500 people aged over 65 years, it appeared that long-term users of anti-inflammatory medication may suffer low rates of ATD. Researchers have suggested that anti-inflammatory medication may play a role in the patho-physiological disease, as markers of inflammation are commonly found at postmortem in patients with the condition (Rozzini, 1996).

Nerve cell degeneration prohibitors or protectors: treatment with nerve growth factor

Synapse degeneration in cortical areas is a well documented feature of early ATD. Drugs influencing cell growth are assumed to be potential inhibitors of this degenerative process. Nerve growth factor stimulates trophic action in the neurons in the developing organism as atrophic processes dominate ATD brains. A lack of one or more trophic factors in these brains might be postulated, but this has not been substantiated. Research continues in treating dementia with intraventricular nerve growth factor. The use of nicotine receptor agonists is also being researched.

Catecholaminergic function stimulation

Drugs that stimulate catecholaminergic function improve cognitive performance. However, the influence of these drugs on memory appears to be attributed mainly to changes in vigilance, arousal and concentration. The monoamine-oxidase β inhibitor selegiline has been shown to cause improvement in patients with ATD (Gottfries, 1994; Lawlor, 1996). Short-term selegiline treatment produced improvement in behaviour and had a significant effect on cognition in patients with ATD, with associated behaviour disturbance.

Hormone replacement therapy

The use of estrogen promotes the growth of cholinergic neurones, stimulates the secretase metabolism of amyloid precursor protein and may interact with apolipoprotein E. Post-menopausal use of the hormone may delay the onset and decrease the risk of ATD in elderly women (Tand, 1996). Long-term, low dose estrogen replacement may improve cognitive function, dementia symptoms and daily activities in women with mild to moderate Alzheimer's dementia (Ohkura, 1995). Literature reviews, however, tend to be poorly focused and unsystematic and there is little evidence based research to support the use of estrogen therapy in preventing and treating dementia.

Vasodilator drugs

Vasodilator drugs have been advocated for use in dementia. In ATD the primary defect is a deficiency of CNS acetylcholine neurotramsission. Cerebral blood flow only falls after the onset of symptoms and this reduction is probably secondary to neuronal loss and it would appear that vasodilators are unlikely to be of value here. Ischaemia is the cause of death in multi-infarct dementia. Studies using vasodilators for this condition are poorly designed, and there is no solid evidence to support their use.

Drugs with vasodilator properties which are being used in chronic cerebral-vascular disease may also, however, have effects unrelated to the vasodilator action. These are often called nootropics and they tend to improve brain metabolism or protect the brain from accumulating toxic effects. The drugs may increase learning and recall by a variety of non-vasodilator mechanisms, Piracetam is an example. However, studies have shown that improvements in cognitive function are small and inconsistent. Vasodilator agents shown to have a statistically significant positive effect on age-related cognitive decline seem to bring benefit to behaviour rather than to cognitive function, and their efficacy seems to be restricted to dementias of vascular origin.

Glial activation limiter

Activation of glial cells leads to neuronal damage and is seen both in ATD and vascular dementia. Propentofylline limits this activation by reinforcing the normal protective actions of the endogenous cell modulator, adenosine, and secondary messengers. Propentofylline is a xanthine derivative, reported to increase cerebral blood flow, prevent cerebral metabolic disorders in anoxia and improve cerebral oedema. Adenosine may act as a neuroprotective agent in brain ischaemia by inhibiting the ischaemia induced by the release of excitotoxic amino acids and also possibly by improving the circulation in the brain. Propentofylline increases extracellular concentrations of adenosine in the ischaemic brain, and also increases cerebral blood flow by dilatation of the cerebrovasculature. The drug appears to improve impaired learning and memory. Reported side effects are minor and transient.

Current studies suggest that it may well prove to have clinical efficacy in the treatment of both primary and degenerative dementias, such as AD and vascular dementia (Saletu, 1991).

Current drug treatment of patients with Alzheimer's disease

Tacrine

Acetylcholine esterase inhibitors (AChEI), ie. tacrine has been shown to reduce memory impairment in patients with AD. With treatment, up to one third of patients who tolerate an effective dose with mild to moderate AD show a statistically significant improvement in memory and associated symptoms, which may last for six months or longer. However, many patients do not respond and the side effects of treatment include a toxic effect on liver function, which limits its usefulness. Patients responding to tacrine produced dose related improvements on objective performance based tests, clinician and care giver related global evaluations and measures of quality of life (Knapp et al, 1994). Tacrine therapy produces elevations in liver enzymes in approximately half of patients with AD. In most cases, elevations will be mild and manageable, and liver enzyme ALT elevations return to normal after tacrine therapy is discontinued. The potential for serious hepatic toxicity can be reduced through careful monitoring of ALT levels in patients who may benefit from tacrine therapy (Watkins et al, 1994).

A proportion of patients with AD will derive some, if modest, benefit from tacrine — particularly if they are able to tolerate the higher doses. Side effects require close supervision and monitoring of patients on treatment (Wilcock, 1994). Other side effects of tacrine treatment are usually of gastrointestinal nature, such as nausea, vomiting and diarrhoea.

Evidence based scientific evidence gives little support to widespread use of tacrine in patients with AD, and the drug is not recommended as part of routine management (Schip, 1997). The long-term safety of tacrine, as with other new products, has yet to be evaluated. One of the other AChE drugs is donepezil.

Donepezil (Aricept)

Donepezil is a specific, highly selective reversible non- competitive inhibitor of AChE. It is more selective for AChE and has a longer duration of inhibitory action than either tacrine or physostigmine. Treatment with donepezil, 5 or 10mg daily, is associated with significant improvements in cognitive function, assessed by the Alzheimer's disease assessment scale — cognitive subscale (ADAS-COG), after fourteen and thirty weeks, and in patients' global function after thirty weeks, compared with placebo, in patients with mild to moderate AD (Rogers, 1996).

The most common adverse event experienced with 5mg per day treatment is gastrointestinal events such as nausea, vomiting, diarrhoea, gastric upset, constipation and dizziness. The main adverse effects appear to be cholinergic and treatment brings improvement in specific mental functions, determined by tests of memory, language and praxis. No hepatotoxicity has been demonstrated after twelve weeks treatment. It appears to have all the beneficial effects of tacrine, with far fewer adverse effects, and is easier in administration in its once a day formulation. Prescription of these drugs requires early and accurate diagnosis of dementia with prompt identification of individuals suffering from mild to moderate dementia.

To date, only the results of the single multicentre randomised control trial have been published. Other large studies are due to be published. The drug is easy to administer and has a favourable side effect profile. It may only have modest benefit on some cognitive measures. Improvement in clinical functional status has yet to be adequately proven, and as yet there is no evidence suggesting that donepezil can improve the quality of life of patients suffering from AD. Donepezil has some effect on brain function. The test used to show this (ADAS-COG) has a range from 0 for normal to 70 for severe impairment. In AD the score deteriorates by about 9–11 points per year. Donepezil appears to reduce the score by about four points — roughly equivalent to the deterioration seen over five months in the average patient. The overall effect appears to be a temporary slowing of the rate of decline in patients with earlier dementia, but with no proven long-term benefit. The underlying disease process appear to remain unaffected.

Exelon

Exelon is a pseudo-irreversible carbamate, AChEI, selective for the central nervous system with regional selectivity within the brain for cortex and hippocampus. In double blind controlled studies, patients treated with Exerol experience significantly less deterioration in cognitive function over a six month period than those administered placebo. Relative to placebo, a significantly high proportion of patients treated with the drug demonstrated a clinically meaningful improvement at six months.

There is strong evidence showing a significant dose response relationship which is virtually linear. Exelon appears to be well tolerated with the majority of adverse events of a gastrointestinal nature. These appear to be mild, transient and resolve on continued treatment. Gastro intestinal events of a minor nature are common to this class of drug and currently no safety reasons have emerged as to why the drug cannot be prescribed for longer term use. Prescription depends largely upon the equation of drug efficacy weighed against costs versus the likelihood of continued cognitive deterioration without treatment and any related drug side effects.

Once licensed the drug promises to be of value in the selective treatment of the symptoms of mild to moderate AD. Response with time and the benefit gained is likely to be variable and patients will have to be cautiously selected and monitored carefully. Titration of drug dose between 3 and 12 mg daily may be appropriate. Exelon is contraindicated in patients with known hypersensitivity to other carbonate derivatives but advanced age is not likely to be a contraindication to therapy.

The global, cognitive, functional, behavioural and neuro-psychiatric response of patients to these new drugs need to be carefully monitored. Drug treatment follow-up is required after four weeks, or sooner, to assess side effects or other problems relating to drug treatment, and again after twelve weeks to determine clinical response to treatment. Long-term follow-up will be necessary at least quarterly. If the patient appears not be benefiting from medication, a trial withdrawal of treatment may be appropriate.

Drug treatment for depression

The co-presentation of depression in dementia must be kept in mind. Depression is a frequent co-morbid syndrome in patients with AD, with an incidence of perhaps 40% (Lazarus et al, 1987). Depression in these patients represents a treatable element of the disease pattern. In one study, 60% of geriatric patients with depression and dementia responded to antidepressive therapy (Ancill, 1989). These studies suggest that between one half and two-thirds of patients with dementia who have depression can be greatly improved with medication. In the absence of any other treatable factors and where dysfunctional behaviour is a presenting problem, depression is often a major underlying cause and the disturbed behaviour will improve as the depression resolves. Depression in patients with AD and or other neurodegenerative dementing disorders is both diagnosable and treatable. Choice of the correct antidepressant may bring a vast improvement in the patient's condition, to the advantage of patient, carer and health professional.

Postmortem studies have shown a relatively severe but variable disturbance of serotonergic metabolism in brain tissue taken from patients with ATD. Selective serotonin re-uptake inhibitors (SSRIs) are effective in the treatment of elderly people with depression (O'Hanlon, 1996). Demented patients without depression may display significant improvement in emotional bluntness, confusion, irritability, anxiety, fear, panic and restless- ness after treatment with these drugs. The SSRIs can be used in elderly patients with cognitive disturbance where there is a dominant element of emotional disturbance.

In the past, tricyclic antidepressants were most commonly used to treat depression. The main adverse effect was postural hypotension, which caused falls in the elderly and anticholinergic confusional states compounded an already complicated picture. The added burden of drugs with anticholinergic properties for those with AD should always be questioned and tricyclics avoided where possible. Drug dose titration is important to avoid side-effects with antidepressants.

The presynaptic SSRIs are beneficial. Fluoxetine is comparatively non-sedative and the serotonergic side-effects, such as anxiety, nausea and diarrhoea, are uncommon at a daily dose of 20mg dose — the initial dosage may be 5mg. It can have an anorexic effect and induce weight loss (Kelsey and Grossberg, 1995). An alternative is fluvoxamine which is less stimulating and is given in an initial dose of 25mg, with maintenance of about 100mg, given at night. Sertraline is another mild stimulating agent given in an initial dose of 25mg.

Lofepramine, a tricyclic drug, has few side-effects, few anticholinergic effects and no antiadrenergic effects, is safe in overdose and is usually non-sedative. It has mild anticholinergic properties in higher therapeutic doses. The dose starts at 70mg daily for the elderly and may be increased to 210mg per day. At low doses these agents can often be dramatically effective. They are certainly worth a trial in patients who are apathetic with marked mental and motor retardation, where there is a suspicion of depression. They should be continued for at least 6 months after recovery to reduce the risk of relapse (Katona and Katona, 1996). Antidepressants may take 4–6 weeks or longer to produce benefit in the elderly.

Drug therapy for behavioural problems

Disturbed behaviour is common in dementia and episodic or persistent delirium is part of the natural history of the disease. Behavioural problems manifest as delusions, hallucinations and disturbances of sleep due to disinhibition, and include aggression and wandering. Depression is understandably common with dementia and the emotional disorder often complicates the dementing process.

Side-effects from psychotropic drugs are a prime cause of agitated behaviour in people with dementia. They can also contribute to cognitive and emotional change (Larson *et al*, 1987). When used in the treatment of dementia, psychotropic drugs are interacting with a nervous system that is already substantially damaged and has defective neurotransmitter systems. Most patients with dementia are also elderly and already at special risk in terms of potential side-effects. Psychotropic drugs often produce behaviour indistinguishable from that due to the dementia, such as akathisia, with extrapyramidal side-effects as well as hypotension. These drugs have often been grossly over-used in the past and are still likely to be given in doses that are too high for elderly patients, or for those with dementia (McGrath and Jackson, 1996).

Antipsychotic or neuroleptic drug use in dementia

Although the practice of using neuroleptic drugs for difficult behaviour associated with dementia is widespread, there is limited evidence of efficacy from double blind placebo controlled trials. A placebo response may occur in two thirds of individuals treated with neuroleptic agents for the control of behavioural disorders in dementia. There are no significant therapeutic differences in response between neuroleptic agents used, nor are there identifiable differences between responders to these agents. A high proportion of people with LBTD are sensitive to neuroleptic agents and a significant number of them will experience a severe reaction. Overall, only 18% of patients identified in a meta analysis of neuroleptic treatment showed benefit over placebo (Schneider et al, 1990).

Effects and adverse reactions

The therapeutic effect of antipsychotic drugs results from blockade of the dopamine receptors in the limbic fore brain and some areas of the cortex. These drugs have inherent properties which cause major side-effects. Many cause drowsiness and somnolence with impairment of psychomotor performance. Those with strong anticholinergic actions, such as thioridazine, can cause an acute confusional state, the so-called, 'atropine psychosis', and add to the disturbance in an already disturbed patient. Neuroleptics may worsen already poor coognitive function (McShane et al, 1997).

Many psychotropic drugs cause extrapyramidal effects, such as:
- parkinsonism — a common occurrence with nearly all neuroleptics, eg. haloperidol and prochlorperazine
- acute dystonic reactions — tonic contraction of the muscles of the neck, shoulders and back
- oculogyric crisis
- tardive dyskinesia — usually a late presentation with characteristic orofacial movements
- akathisia — motor restlessness characterised by agitation and inner tension accompanied by displacing movements such as crossing the legs, rocking to and fro, pacing backwards and forwards.

A major problem with all antipsychotics is the risk of provoking *neuroleptic malignant syndrome*. This comprises a muscular rigidity, autonomic disturbance and hyperpyrexia and can occur at any time during treatment. Haloperidol and trifluoperazine are particularly likely to provoke this syndrome, especially if the dosage is increased to high levels over a day or two. Up to half of those patients who are affected die as a result.

Antipsychotic drugs are likely to disturb thermoregulation with resultant failure of physiological control of body temperature and a concomitant risk of hypothermia in cold climates.

Impairment of vasomotor regulation also brings orthostatic hypotension.

The antipsychotics interact with neuroreceptors controlled by the autonomic nervous system, giving rise to adverse effects such as blurred vision, dry mouth, constipation and urinary retention.

To complicate management even further, these drugs also have cardiovascular effects that result in orthostatic hypotension, tachycardia and depresssion of cardiac muscle contractility and cardiac conduction.

Because of these serious and common potential side-effects, every effort should be made to avoid the prescription of anti-psychotic preparations. When they are considered necessary they should be prescribed in small amounts for a short period, with regular review. The removal of antipsychotic medication from a patient's drug regimen, when a possible diagnosis of dementia is being made, may well result in the symptoms improving or disappearing. Careful consideration of possible causes of the disturbances in behaviour should be made before turning to drug prescription (see Chapter 9).

Randomised controlled trials of psychotropic drug prescription, and drug withdrawal from patients in nursing home settings, have shown that there is no increase in behavioural disturbance in the patients, or evidence of staff distress from this source, when withdrawal has taken place (Senna *et al*, 1994). Carefully designed, placebo-controlled studies have addressed the question of whether antipsychotic drugs control agitation and behavioural disturbance (Barnes *et al*, 1982). Only marginal advantages have been shown when placebo preparations have been used in controlled experiments.

When recourse has to be made to drug use, there appears to be little difference in efficacy between neuroleptics. Practically, it appears that the drugs with prominent muscarinic receptor-blocking activity such as thioridazine do not seem to cause much cognitive impairment if used in low doses.

Haloperidol has been widely used in the treatment of behaviour disturbance in dementing patients by psychiatrists in hospital wards, although it is likely to cause akathisic motor disturbance and later-onset dyskinesias and parkinsonism. Few prescribers seem to appreciate that it is nearly 50 times more potent than thioridazine, and the latter is a much safer drug. Keeping in mind that elderly people are particularly sensitive to extrapyramidal side-effects, these tranquillisers should only be used for disturbed behaviour which defies other management strategies. Thioridazine 10mg three to four times a day is best used with a clearly identifiable role and regular review. An alternative is to identify the time when the disturbed behaviour is maximal; a single dose of the drug given at this time will frequently ameliorate the disturbance. Alternatively, if thioridazine is ineffective, haloperidol 0.25mg can be tried.

Common adverse reations to psychotropic drugs

	Hypotension	Sedation	Extrapyramidal motor disturbance
Thioridazine	Moderate	Severe	Mild
Chlorpromazine	Severe	Severe	Moderate
Haloperidol	Mild	Mild	Severe
Trifluoperazine	Mild	Mild	Severe

Neuroleptics should only be considered for patients:
- with serious problems
- in the presence of serious distress
- showing dangerous problem behaviour
- suffering psychotic symptoms, such as delusions or hallucinations.

Non-drug treatment should always be considered along with drug options before treatment is started. When drug treatment is necessary for confusion, nocturnal wandering and incontinence, short-term clormethiazole instead of thioridazine might be considered with regular review. Where neuroleptic treatment is unavoidable, low doses should be prescribed initially with slow and cautious increases as necessary. The risk of side effects must be taken into acount and balanced against any perceived benefit of medication. Treatment should normally be short-term, with frequent, regular reviews at short intervals. The dose should be reduced as soon as possible, and treatment stopped if it is no longer essential. Routine use of anti-cholinergic medication to prevent extra-pyramidal side effects is not appropriate.

Neuroleptics should normally be avoided where there is a possibility of LBTD.

Non-neuroleptic medication for behavioural disturbance

Non-neuroleptic drugs such as lithium, beta-blockers, anxiolytics and selegiline have been used in the treatment of behavioural disorders. However, their efficacy and safety in modifying behavioural symptoms has been poorly studied, and there is a poor evidence base for their use. Carbamazepine has been used for specific behaviour such as aggression, over-activity, but results of research is equivocal. Trazodone has also been used to reduce agitated behaviour associated with behaviour, and again there is scant evidence of efficacy.

Drug therapy for sleep disturbance

Sleep disturbance, particularly of episodic or persistent night-time wakefulness, is commonly reported in people with dementia. This is usually a major problem for home carers. It may be a symptom of depression and this should be considered and treated where applicable. Many drugs that are commonly used in the management of demented patients can impair sleep. Paradoxically, when demented patients are excessively sedated during the day the effects of drug therapy should be considered.

Persistent disturbed patterns of sleep/wakefulness activity may be best managed by environmental considerations rather than drug medication. Few clinical trials have reported on the efficacy of hypnotic medication in people with dementia. Hypnotics are over-used in nursing homes and in general practice with elderly people, particularly dementing patients. These drugs should always be reviewed regularly and withdrawn at the earliest possible opportunity. If there is marked behavioural disturbance that does not respond to any other approach then a short-acting hypnotic sedative such as clormethiazole can be used. A small dose of thioridazine, 10–25mg at night, may well be effective.

Anxiety disorders and medication

It is hardly surprising that anxiety may be a prominent symptom in the early stages of cognitive degenerative disease. The GP has to be mindful, however, that it may be a symptom of a depressive condition. Stressors ought to be sought and an effort made in counselling in the early stages of the disease, when it is often most needed. Generally, an anxiety state with restlessness and insomnia in those with dementia is more likely to respond to antidepressants or low doses of neuroleptics such as thioridazine, than to the benzodiazepines frequently used in the general population (Salzman, 1990), the latter is frequently associated with falls and hospitalisation (Neutel, 1996). It is wise to search diligently for any environmental causes of anxiety that might be dealt with, before turning to medication.

Confusional states can arise as part of a continuing and dementing process, but they can equally be the result of other conditions. A sudden change in behaviour in the dementing person is likely to be a non-specific presentation of a physical illness. Virtually any illness or drug may induce delirium in a dementing and elderly subject. Urinary tract infection and pneumonia are common precipitants of acute confusional state, as is congestive cardiac failure.

People with structural brain disease, such as AD, have a marked predisposition to the development of delirium, clouding of consciousness, disorientation, delusions, and vivid hallucinations. Fluctuating states of alertness and disturbed sleep/wake patterns should always prompt consideration of whether there is a reversible toxic or metabolic cause affecting the brain and other organs.

Abrupt decline in function with confusion should call for an immediate assessment and review of the patient and current management. It is often wise to withdraw all drugs to see whether the patient improves. Patients' behavioural problems bring GPs into immediate day-to-day management of geriatric patients at home and in nursing homes; for a short time they may become the key worker until these problems have been resolved. At other times they may only be responsible for care team liaison and orchestrating comprehensive medical and social responses to the patient's problems. When it comes to disturbances in behaviour, an appropriate and effective response is vital and should prompt several considerations. Appropriate therapy may:

- help to keep a patient at home

- help the carer to cope a little longer with a difficult situation
- improve quality of life for both patient and carer
- avoid institutionalisation.

An appropriate GP response to behavioural disturbance in a demented patient requires:

1. An overview of environmental features that might cause disturbing behaviour.
2. Reappraisal of the general situation in terms of carer and care input.
3. Review/reassessment of the patient's physical status.
4. A diligent search for coexisting treatable conditions.

In the last extreme, drug medication may be appropriate and very effective, but in terms of hypnotics, anxiolytics, antidepressants and anti-psychotics they should be used in low dose, in the short-term and mindful of adverse side-effects.

Treatment of vascular dementia

Unlike ATD, vascular dementia is preventable. There is evidence that controlling the vascular risk factors, such as hypertension, diabetes and hypercholesterolaemia, can improve cognitive function (Amar and Wilcock, 1996).

Hypotensive and lipid-lowering agents should therefore be considered in treatment, and good control of diabetes should be maintained.

Anticoagulation with warfarin in patients with atrial fibrillation will rarely be appropriate because of the risk from falls and poor compliance. However, antiplatelet treatment with low-dose aspirin, 75mg daily, should be considered.

Those with substantial carotid stenosis should be considered for surgery.

Patients who have primary cerebral systemic vasculitis with secondary brain involvement may benefit from immuno-suppressive drugs such as corticosteroids.

Aspirin therapy

Reduction in risk of further vascular events, for people with early dementia known to be related to cerebral ischaemia, may be achieved by treatment with aspirin, 75mg daily. The magnitude of any effect on cognitive impairment is unclear, but stroke is a significant risk factor in the development of vascular dementia (North England Guideline Project, 1997).

Hydergine

Reviews and studies of hydergine, a vasodilator, demonstrate small cognitive improvements of variable sustainability. Responders to the drug can not be predicted in advance. Hydergine is not considered sufficiently effective to be routinely recommended.

Hydergine has been prescribed for dementia for the past five decades. However, several placebo-controlled studies have not been able to substantiate any clear-cut benefit from the use of this product (Thompson *et al*, 1990).

Multi-infarct dementia has been called a 'preventable senility' and hypertension is a major risk factor for this disorder. The Framingham study (Farmer *et al*, 1987), however, suggested that high blood pressure was linked to improved psychometric test scores in subjects over 75 years of age. In younger age groups, vascular changes may be more important causes of cognitive decline than the changes of AD. There may well be a case for treating the under-75s who have hypertension and cognitive impairment with hypotensive agents. Calcium-channel blockers may also improve focal brain ischaemia and limit excitotoxicity, but further work remains to be done in this field.

9
Non-drug interventions in dementia management

Little is known about how individuals adapt emotionally and cognitively to degenerative dementia, therefore psychological, behavioural and family interventions are poorly developed. Established therapeutic techniques should, however, be utilised (Goldsmith, 1996). The general principles of management should be appreciated by the GP. Most of the management will fall to a delegated nurse or other professional carer, but it is the responsibility of the GP to ensure that optimal management is provided and that the delegated professional is aware of good practice, treatment options, and the local support facilities and resources available. The Stirling University Dementia Services Development Centre (DSDC) has produced a valuable guide for community nurses working in the dementia field (Archibald *et al*, 1995). This guide emphasises that:

1. In general, recourse to drug medication should be avoided.
2. The specific causes of the behaviour should be sought and an endeavour made to alter unacceptable conduct by removing or altering the behavioural triggers.
3. The circumstances in which the behaviour occurs should be considered. It may be that environmental change, such as quieter, calmer surroundings, will bring about improvement.

Efforts should concentrate on seeking a means of returning the patient to more normal and acceptable behaviour and endeavour to reduce the excess load on the carer resulting from the patient's unacceptable behaviour. This may mean building in respite care, so that carers can distance themselves physically from the disturbing situation for a recognised period of time.

Professional health carers should focus on seeking an explanation for the disturbed behaviour, and then try to interpret and understand it, before responding with an individualised careplan. Improving communication with the patient is a vital prerequisite and the communication process is an important ingredient in the promotion of good dementia care.

Coping with difficult problems

People with dementia who live in the community usually have some degree of cognitive functioning remaining. Although the extent of brain function will be variable, there is a residual rationality in many of these people. Even the most impaired often have preferences. The key to much dementia management revolves around communication, which is understandably complex when one considers the many communication skills that are lost in the dementing process.

Automatic language skills, such as saying 'Hello' in return to a greeting, and habitual responses that are said without thinking, are retained for the longest time. Aspects of communication that require careful thought are soon lost. Generally, people with dementia communicate feelings, and they do this symbolically in a non-verbal fashion. It is this behaviour that has to be interpreted in order to understand what patients are endeavouring to communicate.

People with dementia also appear to be particularly tuned to the non-verbal information that we communicate ourselves. Doctors who have developed neurolinguistic programming skills, currently seen as a means of improving the patient/doctor interaction, are well placed to appreciate non-verbal interaction. Other health care givers may have to be educated towards a similar approach. Another key to communication in people with dementia is knowledge of the person's past, which is often well known to the family doctor but a closed book to other health care providers. When speaking to people with dementia, messages must be sent to them which they can understand. A few simple guidelines will help to improve difficult communication.

Any communication barriers deserve attention. Efforts should be made to diminish or remove obstacles to understanding. This will promote better management and improved behaviour in the patient.

Barriers to good communication with people with dementia:

Competing input	–	distractions such as television or the radio
Sensory defects	–	age-related defects in vision and hearing
Attitudes	–	the patient may have no insight
Memory deficit	–	affects concentration and conversation flow

Confusion	–	the patient may be confused.
Disorientation	–	the patient is disoriented in time and place
Poor attention span	–	inability to concentrate
Comfort status	–	if the patient is physically uncomfortable, eg. needing to toilet, he/she may be preoccupied and unable to concentrate
Dysphasia	–	receptive and expressive problems

Communication barriers — carer with patient

Examples of communication barriers between carer and patient are:
- carer's lack of background knowledge of the patient
- carer's rigid professional views regarding behaviour and the illness
- unhelpful attitudes such as: patient is mad; cannot be helped; frightening; dangerous; should be in hospital; isn't my problem.

Communication can be improved by both verbal and non-verbal imput

Verbal input

Volume	–	speak loudly and clearly; avoid shouting
Speed	–	allow time for the patient to understand the content
Tone of voice	–	speak in normal tones; do not use baby talk
Appropriate choice of words	–	keep sentences short and only proffer one piece of information at a time; use experience to bridge past and present
Prompt	–	prompts can act as a reminder, eg. identifies the person, the day of the week
Questions	–	avoid open questions, eg. 'What would you like to eat?'; be more specific, eg. 'Would you like fish?'
Content	–	avoid implied messages

Non-verbal input

Eye contact	–	face the person and establish contact
Personal intrusion	–	be aware of personal space; stand close, but not too close, facing the person, within their line of vision. Capture their attention
Facial expressions	–	enhance communication; they may be incongruous, eg. inappropriate expressions for content of speech
Gestures	–	use your own hands and arms to communicate; consider the meaning of the patient's gestures
Physical contact	–	a gentle touch helps to alleviate anxiety; however, physical contact can sometimes be experienced as a threat
Environment	–	avoid distracting noises or interruption

Professional carers should develop awareness of communication problems which beset the patient. Environmental factors can play a prominent part in affecting the quality of communication. Location, time of day, background noises, competing distractions and general fatigue should all be considered, and the background manipulated, if possible, to provide a good communicative milieu. Good management of disruptive behaviour involves finding out why people are behaving in a certain way, which assumes that there are reasons for the behaviour. If these can be found, something may be done to change the behaviour. Many GPs are undertaking courses on neurolinguistic programming to improve their communication skills. These can be valuable in helping GPs to understand the problems that people with dementia experience in thinking.

Neurolinguistic programming

Neurolinguistic programming is the study of how language and the cognition of external events affect our behaviour. Language in this context includes the visual, auditory, kinaesthetic, olfactory and gestatory senses and 'self-talk'. The senses shape, form and limit what is perceived, with experience filtering in and out the input, to make it consistent with expectations. An internal representation of the world map is created and people act and communicate in response to perceived events.

In dementia, the thinking processes are distorted and sensory input is misinterpreted, so that the demented person's internal map of the world is not the same as the normal individual's perception of it. Patients' behaviour can provide clues as to how they have put their map together. The health professional's task is to expand ways in which they can make sense of their world. Improved communication requires attention to all the non-verbal language modalities. Better communication will bring better understanding of the patient's difficulties, the opportunity to help the patient overcome them, and improvement in challenging behaviour.

Psychosociological methods of care management

These therapies have proved difficult to evaluate and they do have their critics (Roth, 1996). At the very least, they offer something to combat therapeutic nihilism, which is still met with in the care of this group of patients. The GP should be aware of such therapies and their potential and be prepared to encourage their use by the carer and members of the primary care team.

Reality orientation and reminiscence are commonly used techniques, with the former being used informally in one-to-one interactions. The basic concept is that inaccuracies made by the person with the illness should be confronted and *reality orientation* provides visual and verbal cues which help mitigate the disorientation that can accompany dementia (Morton and Bleathman, 1991). It is believed that the approach improves verbal orientation and the quality of interaction between carer and the person with the illness.

Reminiscence work is based on the notion of life review, which permits old people to make sense of and resolve past conflicts. It involves the use of a variety of personalised aids that prompt memory, reaffirm a sense of self and have relevance for that particular person. There is some evidence that reminiscence therapy improves mood (Goldwasser et al, 1987).

Validation therapy challenges the basic concepts of reality orientation by focusing on the affirmation of, rather than a confrontation with, the person's sense of reality by assuming that patient behaviour and speech have an underlying meaning. The carer 'validates' the patient's conversation by attention to the emotional rather than the factual content. There is evidence that stimulating therapeutic activities help to reduce the patient's frustration levels (Rovner et al, 1996).

Validation therapy is believed to:
- restore a feeling of self-worth in the patient
- increase verbal and non-verbal communication
- prevent inward withdrawal
- reduce stress
- decrease the need for medication (Klerk, 1994).

While the efficacy of validation therapy has been poorly evaluated, both family and professional carers can employ these techniques. However, changes in orientation and self-care can only be promoted and maintained with continuous input from carers. Strategies have to be tailored to the individual with a goal-planning approach for each individual patient as the objective. The attending doctor should be aware of these techniques and be prepared to encourage the nurse or other professional carer to utilise them or, alternatively, ensure that the patient has access via a clinic or day centre. Many family carers are prepared to take some of these concepts on board, as it makes them feel that they are doing something personally to help the individual concerned cope with the dementia.

The family doctor should be aware of these psychological approaches, if only to ensure that they have been considered or put in place by the key worker. The GP may have to educate and stimulate the nurse or other health worker to consider these techniques and incorporate them within therapeutic objectives. Many family carers are pleased to be involved in such a therapeutic programme, which obviously has to be tailored to the individual and the stage of the illness.

Rehabilitation and care management are about being positive, searching for things that patients can do for themselves and enabling them to do so. It is about looking forward, cooperating with patients and encouraging them in what they can do. In essence, the nurse's role is about enabling and facilitating and, if necessary, trying to recapture motivation (Royal College of Nursing, 1991). The patient with developing dementia should not be deprived of this attention just because his/her cognitive deficit makes communication difficult.

Expressive therapies such as physical exercise, visual art and music appear to decrease problem behaviours (Beck et al, 1992). It has been suggested that the observed functional decline in dementing illnesses may be as much a function of the social care received as of the biological causes (Gilhooley et al, 1994). It is felt that supportive environments can prolong independence, encourage self-reliance and improve the quality of life for people with dementia. *Activity programmes* designed specifically for persons with dementia have been developed and promote sensory stimulation, exercise, reminiscence, socialisation and self-esteem (Zgola, 1990).

Reality orientation

Reality orientation (Holden, 1990) led the way in drawing attention to the possibility that people with dementia could learn and could be helped to adjust to reality. This has now led to an increased focus on intervention techniques such as validation therapy (Feil, 1982). Reality orientation developed as a means of orientating a person to their locale by the use of procedures that try to keep confused persons in touch with personal facts and their environment. Often done in small group therapy, the technique consists of repeatedly presenting the facts of orientation, eg. time, date and place, to patients with positive reinforcement and encouragement. It can work quite well with patients who are withdrawn and therefore not using their remaining faculties to the full, and also in those who lack confidence. In terms of scientific validity its efficacy is still debated, but there is evidence that it is partly effective over short periods for some people, and it generally has a stimulating effect on the patients. It is still believed by many to have a therapeutic place in current management (Holden, 1990) and stimulates patients into relearning things about themselves and their environment.

Twenty-four hour reality orientation is a term used to describe efforts in nursing and residential homes to maintain communication with the dementia sufferer through their daily living cycle by restructuring the personal environment in the hope of improving orientation, and by communication through use of recurrent reminders, eg. their name, events of the day, etc. It can be promoted by simple changes in the physical environment such as installing clocks, calendars, and talking clocks. Some demented people can perceive symbols better than words. The use of both words and pictures may help them, eg. in determining the whereabouts of the toilet. Family carers and professional staff remind the patient repeatedly of their orientation and endeavour to correct any disorientation. Again, orientation aids can help by simple labelling of rooms or objects. Patients are directed to the aids, asked to read them, and reminded of their association. This requires staff and carer commitment and involves gently reminding the patient of present reality and correcting mistaken ideas, with the patient actively involved in working out issues. In reality orientation the patient is the focus of attention and the technique encourages verbal orientation and functioning. It does not work with those who are confused, rambling and wandering. There is evidence that dementia patients can learn new information, although at a slower rate than normal (Morris and Baddeley, 1988).

Reminiscence therapy

This type of therapy is also used (Butler, 1963). It encourages the patient to think and talk about past experience through the use of memorabilia, pictures and slides. Psychologists and occupational therapists believe it capitalises on remaining function and preserves it. It helps patients to focus on positive past memories. With instruction, family carers can adopt some of these methods. Reminiscence therapy has no clear focus, but it can be used as an interaction activity and can improve orientation when used with reality orientation.

Reminiscence therapy has been said to use the 'then and there' of life to enrich the 'here and now' (Goldsmith, 1996). It has several advantages. It helps to:
- develop relationships with carers
- maintain self-esteem
- preserve self-identity
- give feelings of belonging to society
- relay history and wisdom to the young
- promote therapeutic support by encouraging resolution, re-organisation and re-integration of the patient's past life-events (Murphy, 1994).

As one patient has recorded:

'His tuntra'd mind sprouts leaflets here and there
and causes me to stare,
in new awareness of the man
he must have been.

> *Where he now struggles to retain
> such meagre lichen to his brain
> he must have raised rare orchids
> in years long seen.'*

(Davis, 1989)

This procedure involves looking back into the patient's past with their co-operation. Patients usually have recall of long past life events and reminiscence allows people to recall the significance of their past, and their status as a real person in the real world. It also helps professional carers to appreciate the patient's former standing in the community, and encourages respect for them as people with human status. The creation of a life book with old photographs, newspaper cuttings and memorabilia at the onset of the dementing process can be a useful aid in later therapy. The process will sometimes reveal parts of working memory that are still relatively untouched by the dementing process, eg. singing. The patient can be encouraged to explore this avenue of communication. An aphasic person may still be able to vocalise in song.

Validation therapy

Validation therapy was developed as a more sensitive and empathetic procedure than reality orientation (Feil, 1982). Validation has its strength in recognising that whatever words the patient uses and whatever feelings they have are in fact true, and carers can respond to them without fear of promoting further confusion. Empathy and understanding are associated with validation, and procedures work primarily on a cognitive feeling level. Validation has been defined as an empathetic approach, affirming the personal reality of the demented person. The validation method describes stages of progressive disorientation and defines specific techniques that can be used at each stage. It encourages care givers — both professional and family — to accept that patients' cognitive losses cannot be retrieved but can be helped along the path from whatever point they have reached. This technique is not useful in disorientated patients.

Recreational activities

Exercise has protective effects in decreasing mortality and is associated with decreased disability and risk of myocardial infarction. It is also very effective in the very old (Elon, 1996). The Dementia Services Development Centre, Stirling University has produced several books on the practical aspects of therapeutic activities for people with dementia (Archibald, 1990).

Cognitive deficiency and behavioural problems

The ability to use and manipulate language is a primary element of social interaction. Loss of cognitive skills can blight social communication. Cognitive decline is not synonymous with advancing age, but is associated with age-related diseases; atherosclerosis results in a considerable increase in the proportion of cognitively impaired older people (Breteler *et al*, 1992). Cognitive skills are controlled by the cerebral cortex. They are specifically affected by organic disease such as dementia. Disturbed thinking processes do not intermesh with the normal thinking responses of the carer, resulting in failure in two-way communication.

Cognitive deficiencies occur in acquiring and manipulating knowledge, and affected individuals display shortfalls in attention, memory, language, imagery, reasoning and perception. Deficiencies in these cognitive skills vary markedly with the severity of the disease and some intellectual skills decline more speedily than others. Patients start progression through the dementing process from different levels of function, and losses will be variable, interact and mean different things at different times. Loss of connections between different brain functions result in disconnection, which itself interferes with many cognitive functions.

Loss of skills can affect:
- the receipt, processing and storing of information
- expression of communication
- initiation of the functional response.

There is also a loss of control over input to the brain and output from the brain, with further problems from neurological disinhibition.

In some instances, cognitive losses can result in *paranoid delusions* which can be difficult for carer and professionals to deal with. Emotional disinhibition also occurs and there is emotional lability and *stuck emotions*. The emotions can change with great rapidity, so that the patient can be showing signs of depression one moment and be wildly euphoric the next — this is known as *emotional incontinence.* In many instances, stuck emotions can appear as a flattening of affect which may be interpreted by the doctor as a form of depression. Sometimes the patient will have retained insight and be embarrassed by these actions. An extreme form of emotional inhibition is called *catastrophic reaction;* this may occur during the assessment process or at times when the patient is apparently overloaded with a complicated mental problem beyond his/her resources to contain.

Disinhibition of speech results in *perseveration* when the individual has difficulty shifting from one subject to another. It is rare for people without any form of brain disease to demonstrate perseveration, which is therefore a useful sign in recognising dementia. It often occurs when orientation, memory and other brain function are normal. *Stuck speech,* where the individual repetitively enunciates the same word or phrase, is common in people with dementia — this has been called the *gramophone sign.*

Loss of control over brain input can affect attention and dementing patients are incapable of focusing attention for any length of time and are easily distracted. However, in some instances they also exhibit *stuck attention* when attention gets fixed on one object, and they become engrossed in that sound or sight.

Disturbances in information reception, processing and storage

Incoming information is affected by loss of perception, attention and concentration.

Processing the information is adversely affected by lack of motivation, personality disturbance, affective disturbance and the speed of thinking, fantasising and problem solving.

Information storage depends on memory which is badly disturbed in short-term stores. Disturbance of information storage also affects new learning capacity and expression of speech, with problems in enunciating speech and co-ordinating appropriate responses.

Failure of brain function results in the loss of control over brain input and output, with resultant disinhibition and behavioural upset. *Defective brain input* results in an inability to maintain attention, hallucinations and delusions. *Upset to brain output* results in disinhibition in speech, emotions, thinking, planning and behaviour.

Neurological disinhibition in dementia can result in incontinence, usually of urine, although some patients also demonstrate faecal incontinence. Family and professional carers find these problems the hardest to cope with. Not only is there chronic incurable illness but there are also new behaviour patterns not previously associated with the individual concerned. Different losses and different degrees of loss have considerable practical significance in terms of the problems they create for the carer.

Management of these deficits often depends on:
- identifying the deficit
- recognising what the patient is still capable of doing
- endeavouring to replace what is missing
- maximising the residual skills.

Although many of the interconnections between the cerebral functions may have been lost, the patient will have retained other connections which may have been little used in the past, but which are available if tapped and utilised. This often requires management involving patient stimulation, to encourage retention and extension of the person's usage of remaining cortical functions. For instance, some patients who have become aphasic after stroke retain the capacity to sing, and if this is appreciated the skill can be used by the therapist in rehabilitation.

Cognitive disinhibition

The effects of cognitive disinhibition are generally worse in the early stages of dementia and tend to lessen as the dementia progresses and becomes severe. Self-control has been part of a learning process developed over many years. It involves the frontal lobes which control functions such as conscience, judgment, morality and social awareness. The loss of these social controls can be quite an early problem in dementia, and is sometimes the first sign to be picked up by the carer.

Clinical presentation of cognitive losses

Losses present as minor failures in judgment, cleanliness, manners, conversation and dressing, but these can be major practical problems for those dealing with the individual, especially when they involve exhibition, restlessness, loss of respect for other people's possessions and attention seeking. People with dementia often hold odd ideas as a result of disinhibition of thinking, ideas that contradict each other and ideas that become fixed/delusions. These delusions cannot be shifted by reasoning.

Visual hallucinations can also be a problem. However, they are more frequently evidence of delirium and a cause for this should be sought. Detection of hallucinations can be difficult and depends on the patient's account of the experiences and what he/she makes of them.

Loss of brain function and control is often the cause of the *behavioural problems* which most frequently disturb the carer and involved health professional. An understanding of their cause and efforts to relieve underlying problems are an essential part of management. Treatment may be the responsibility of the carer or attending nurse, but it is important that the GPs are aware of the available techniques and treatments so that they can educate carers/nurses or point them towards individuals who can help them. The doctor can ensure input from occupational therapists, speech and language therapists or other health professionals to help minimise the effects of cognitive losses in dementing patients. Occasionally appropriate drug medication may help to alleviate these disturbances.

10
Management of challenging behaviour

Problem behaviours

Disruptive features exhibited by people with dementia (Rapp *et al*, 1992) include the following:

Feature	% of patients affected
Agitation	85
Wandering	60
Depression	60
Screaming	25
Violence	20

The ABC technique is often used in coping with challenging behaviour:

A	—	What is the activating event?
	—	What precedes the disruptive behaviour?
B	—	What behavioural response has been generated?
C	—	What are the consequences of the behaviour?

Is the person trying to communicate something by exhibiting this behaviour? This question of attempted communication may be the most important element to consider.

Agitation

Agitation may occur in 85% of patients with dementia. It has been defined as inappropriate verbal and vocal or motor activity, which is not explained by the person's apparent needs or current state of

123

confusion. Three agitation syndromes have been described, depending on the primary manifestations:
1. Physical
2. Verbal
3. Disruptive motor function, without (1) or (2).

Overreaction

Dementing patients often react to trivial situations or minor criticism by screaming, shouting and displaying unacceptable vocal behaviour. They tend to become very agitated or refuse to move. **Catastrophic reactions** refer to grossly exaggerated responses that are completely inappropriate to the trigger. A calm, quiet environment makes these reactions less likely and too great a demand should not be made on the patient in terms of questions and tasks.

Anger and hostility

Aggression may be exhibited by 20% of people with dementia. This should be perceived by the carer as a normal reaction to the losses imposed by the disease on the individual. Aggression is often the result of frustration or insecurity, driven by the individual's loss of control over his/her day-to-day life. Loss of ability to express feelings and anxieties mean that these emotions are bottled up and explosions of ill temper may occur. Some of these may be driven by fear and the attending doctor should always consider whether the patient may be the recipient of physical or verbal abuse. Prevention is preferable to having to cope with aggression in a crisis intervention situation: a calm environment, a limited number of demands on the patient, avoidance of confrontation, and a behaviourist approach to establish patterns of behaviour causality are recommended.

Calm and constant routines without excess stimulation should be instituted. Reality orientation may help to reduce excessive behavioural response. It is wise to reinforce the remaining capabilities of the dementing patient and not just focus on disabilities.

The importance of environment

People with dementia are acutely sensitive to their social and physical environment. Their behaviour and wellbeing depend as much on where they are and the way they are being treated as they do on the disease process and medication (Marshall, 1994). A calm, soothing, pleasant milieu can comfort and quieten the most aggressive patient. Attention to the social and physical environs may reduce challenging behaviour without recourse to drug therapy. Quiet, comfort and warmth and reduction of stimulation overload in a person with limited coping ability are prerequisites to good care. Excess noise, heat, cold, light or darkness and lack of personal space or freedom of movement are all disturbing features which can be controlled with forethought (Tooth, 1995).

Coping with aggression

Do not	Do
Confront	Stay calm
Shout or raise voice	
Threaten	
Touch	Avoid invading person's personal space
Attempt physical control	
Physically restrain	
Approach rapidly, especially from behind	Allow the patient environmental space
Take personal offence	Reassure
Ridicule	Listen
	Encourage to talk
Show fear, alarm, anxiety	Divert attention
Corner person, crowd in	Seek additional support from known carer
Provoke a catastrophic reaction	

Wandering

Wandering is a common problem, affecting up to 60% of dementia patients, and is one of the most challenging behavioural problems in dementia. Although there are no absolute solutions, careful observation and thoughtful intervention can reduce the incidence of wandering or remove the need for it (Allan, 1994a).

To wander means to ramble or move with no definite objective. However, patients with dementia who wander often have underlying reasons for this behaviour, although they may themselves be unable to work them out. The liability to wander away from home or to reach some objective destination is a frequent feature of dementia. The fear of wandering and the risk to the wanderer make this a major social concern for family carers and wandering is often the reason for seeking institutional care for a person with dementia. Underlying causes for the behaviour should be sought.

Reasons for wandering (Marshall, 1993):

- boredom — absence of activities to keep person mentally or physically occupied
- loneliness — the search for companionship
- searching — for relative, friend, dead spouse or toilet
- separation anxiety — generated as a result of some other person's actions
- forgetfulness — forgetting purpose of walk
- disorientation — likely to occur when moving between sibling homes, day centres and institutional care
- pottering — no task, no *raison d'être*
- at night time — insomnia. Disorientation in time
- checking and trailing — fear of losing support
- a need for exercise
- expression of anxiety, anger or stress
- a continuation of life style patterns
- a desire to escape the current environment
- failure in navigational skills
- faulty goal-directed behaviour
- side-effect of medication
- concurrent physical or psychological disturbance, eg. a pain from a physical condition being deflected on to other activity or a chronic constipation during a need to find a toilet.

Is the wandering due to short-term memory loss or is the individual just walking about in an extension of pre-illness behaviour? Wandering can be a way of using up excess energy in those accustomed to walking distances when younger or before being overtaken by the illness. It may also be an expression of boredom. Any source of agitation may cause people to pace up and down or to wander off for no apparent reason. There may also be new perceptual problems, resulting in patients failing to recognise their own home. A common, but frequently overlooked, cause of wandering is pain and discomfort which upsets the patient, who is then unable to communicate the problem. Such a problem may often be caused by constipation, or more generalised pains common to the elderly such as arthritis. Other reasons for wandering are disorientation in time or place, and the patient's mistaken belief that he/she should be somewhere else.

There always has to be a degree of compromise in acceptance of personal risk in terms of trauma from falls and separation from the home environment as a result of wandering and restriction of individual freedom and the person's need to move freely about the local milieu. Questions to be considered include:

- is the behaviour prompted by an underlying treatable condition?
- does the person have urinary problems?
- does the person have constipation or a bowel disturbance?
- is he/she disorientated in time or place?
- will orientation aids improve the situation?

People who wander should be provided with an identification bracelet to be worn at all times. The use of restraining chairs, clip-on tables and other physical restraints is condemned as they are a denial of personal liberty and dignity. There are now a number of electronic aids available for monitoring patients who wander and this may be the way forward in the future for people living in the community.

If the source of the wandering cannot be discovered or the behaviour altered, thioridazine 25mg at night for nocturnal wandering, or 10mg during the day before the wandering usually occurs, can be useful. A review of current medication is always advisable when patients begin to wander, as many hypnotics, antipsychotics and other drugs can cause confusion and encourage this type of behaviour.

Cognitive impairment is an independent risk factor for serious injury during falls (Tinetti et al, 1995).

Mental restlessness linked with physical restlessness may be related to a feeling of being lost and not belonging. People have a right to explore their environment and their freedom should not be unduly curtailed.

The pattern of wandering, including time of day and route should be studied and an endeavour made to understand why the wandering is taking place. Drug therapy should be reviewed to ascertain whether this may be the source of the trouble. Controlled removal of medications may be needed to ensure that they are not causing behavioural change.

Management of wandering can be summarised as follows:

1. Seek the cause.
2. Drug review is mandatory.
3. Institute measures to counteract lack of exercise and boredom which encourage wandering.
4. Avoid the use of physical and chemical restraints if at all possible.

Nocturnal wandering is particularly trying for family carers, because it often results in disturbance of sleep for carers who are wakened in the early hours. Some believe that wandering is a myth and that the emphasis should be on the fact that demented people are likely to walk about; that there are reasons for why they do so, and that these should be sought by professional carers (Marshall, 1993).

Questions to consider when seeking the underlying cause of wandering are shown in Figure 10.1.

Sundowning is the term used for confusion, that often occurs in the late afternoon or early evening when there is a tendency for the patient to walk about and wander. It can be caused by drug medication, or by dehydration if the patient is not eating or drinking properly.

It is not delirium (Bliwise, 1994) and it is not unique to dementing patients as it occurs in other forms of brain disease.

Insomnia and disturbed sleep are very common in people with dementia, often becoming more marked in the middle or later phases of the disease. There is disturbance in the sleep/wake cycle. Frequently, getting off to sleep presents no problem but there is wakening in the early hours with a distinct possibility that the patient will be disorientated in time and place and may wander. Again the cause of the change in behaviour has to be sought. Sometimes the change in behaviour is due to inappropriate drug medication, or people sleeping too much during the day. On other occasions it may be due to urinary

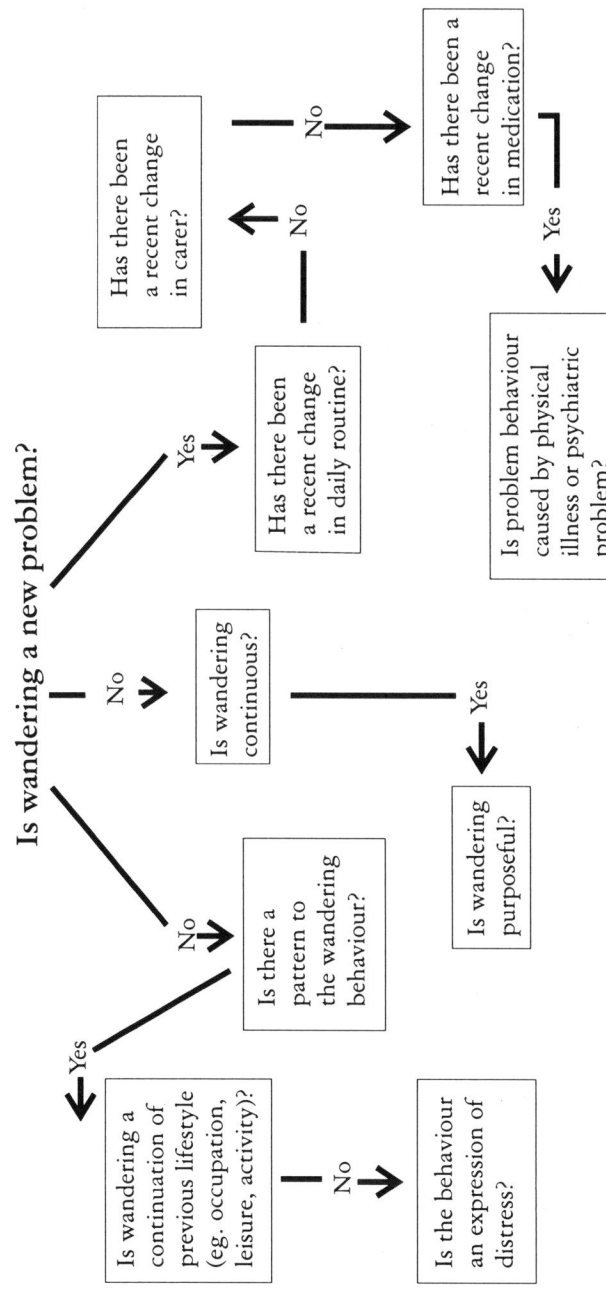

Figure 10.1: Questions to be considered when seeking the cause of wandering behaviour

tract infection with resulting need to toilet during the night. It may also be caused by pain or depression.

This feature can be particularly distressing to family carers already overstretched by the demands of day care. The disturbed nights are likely to undermine the carers' health and they are also likely to fear that patients may wander out of the house, unbeknown to the sleeping carers. If the difficulty in sleeping is due to depression the pattern may be inability to fall asleep with early morning waking.

Withdrawn behaviour can be due directly to the progression of the dementia, but is equally likely to be precipitated by depression. The possibility of patient abuse has also to be kept in mind with the patient's conduct a response to physical and verbal abuse. Depression occurs in 40–60% of dementing patients and may cause a retreat into isolation or withdrawal (Liston, 1978). Withdrawal may also result from a fear of failure in carrying out normal activities of daily living and a concern about loss of control, and communication skills. Withdrawal is often a sign of the patient's internal distress and need for counselling.

Patients should have their physical condition checked, medication reviewed and behaviour assessed, including psychological appraisal. Assessment should also consider the patient's interpersonal relationship with members of the family to exclude patient abuse. Insomnia and altered sleep patterns may be evidence of depression. Where there is no overt physical cause, a 6-week trial of a low dose of serotonin re-uptake inhibitor is justifiable, provided that its prescription is carefully monitored for side-effects. This medication can be remarkably effective in covert depression and often brings a prompt improvement in mood, motivation and socialisation within a week or two of initiation of treatment.

Urinary and faecal incontinence

Incontinence should prompt a search for specific causes such as pain, the need for toileting, lack of daytime exercise, excessive day-time sleeping, constipation.

Management involves:
- exclusion of urinary tract infection
- exclusion of vaginal and perineal infection in women
- exclusion of diabetes mellitus
- anticipation of toilet needs

- regulated routine of daytime activities, rest and exercise
- treatment of depression or pain
- review of medications for side-effects
- avoidance of beverages containing caffeine and heavy meals late in the evening; avoidance of too many caffeine-containing drinks such as coffee and cola during the day
- establishment of consistent bedtime rituals and discouragement of daytime napping.

A framework for tackling incontinence is shown in Figure 10.2.

Urinary incontinence is distressing for patient and carer and often a driving force in determining institutionalisation (Argyll, 1985). Incontinence may be one aspect of the natural progression of Alzheimer's disease. However, it is frequently concomitant to the existing condition and there should be prompt treatment of urinary tract infection, constipation, uncontrolled diabetes, enlarged prostrate, vaginitis. Review of diuretics should also be made. In the absence of treatable infection, three hourly toileting after meals and before bedtime on a regular basis may well contain the problem. Reducing fluid intake after 4.00 pm can help and incontinence pads should be prescribed and a laundry service organised if it becomes a chronic problem.

Management of urinary incontinence

Cause	Management
Urinary tract infection	Midstream specimen of urine Antibiotic
Vaginitis	Vaginal swab Antibiotic
Constipation	Rectal examination Proctoscopy Manual removal of faeces if necessary Appropriate diet
Failure to recognise the toilet	Use of orientation aids

Diuretics	Review and reduce dose
	Change drug
Stress incontinence	Physical examination
	Refer to gynaecologist
Bladder dysfunction	Refer to urologist
Loss of control which remains unresponsive to intervention	Incontinence aids, eg. Urosheaths, pads, therapy, Kanga pads

These causes of urinary incontinence demand the same attention as they would when occurring with any elderly patient. However, people with dementia may have additional difficulties because of their memory impairment and disorientation in finding the toilet, with resulting incontinence. Additional sign posting in the house may help, and a regular toileting programme should be instituted. Patients with poor memory may have to be regularly routed to the toilet in a relearning exercise.

The incontinence of dementia is a neurological phenomenon, as the patient usually has a normal bladder but there is a disinhibition of messages from the diseased frontal lobes of the brain. Spinal cord messages are interrupted on the way to the bladder, and the patient's bladder opens when it reaches a certain size and pressure — with the patient unaware of the problem. Retraining can be useful if incontinence is of recent onset. The patient needs regular reminders that he/she may need the toilet, and praise for making a successful toilet journey. Regular 2-3-hourly toileting can re-institute continence, with reinforcement. Antispasmodic drugs, such as flavoxate, can be tried. They often work for a remarkably long time despite the steady physical deterioration associated with dementia.

In many instances the dementia progresses to a total loss of urinary and sometime faecal continence. At this point incontinence aids such as special absorbent pads will be required, and patient and carer should be encouraged to take advantage of the free laundry service. Ultimately, an indwelling catheter may have to be considered. However, these devices are not always well tolerated by patients who tend to fiddle with them and pull them out. Faecal incontinence brings an inevitable request for the patient to be institutionalised. In early dementia, faecal incontinence is usually just a sign of simple constipation. Rectal examination, laxative administration, and manual evacuation of faeces may be required to solve the problem. Faecal incontinence may also result from drug side-effects and the drug regimen should be reviewed.

Falls

Dementia is an important risk factor for falling (Takashi, 1996). Falls in the elderly result in fractures of the neck of the femur and are associated with institutionalisation and an increased mortality.

Falls are also associated with significant morbidity. They are more likely to occur if there is a history of falling in the last year, and if the patient is on medication, eg. antipsychotics, diuretics, antihypertensives, cardiotonics, hypnotics and sedatives.

In people with dementia the frequency of falling increases because of misperception of environmental dangers and loss of cognition. Wandering and agitated behaviour increase the risk of a fall.

Patients with dementia who have a history of falls merit the same assessment and investigation of causes as any other elderly person. Management should include a careful drug review to exclude side-effects as the cause of falls as well as considering the presence of:

- infection
- arthritis
- transient ischaemic attacks
- episodes of acute confusion
- hypoglycaemia
- dehydration
- anaemia.

Behavioural management techniques

Behavioural management techniques focus on the individual patient by trying to understand the person in relation to the environment. Unacceptable behaviours can be related to objects and specific situations. These methods do not claim to eliminate a particular problem entirely, but they often highlight causes which can then be addressed. Such techniques are based on observation and are effective for inappropriate sexual behaviour, wandering, aggression and incontinence. Many people with dementia are highly stressed, and this can impair their functioning and be a cause of wandering and agitation (Marshall, 1993).

The use of behaviour management techniques to treat presentations of challenging behaviour involve a study of mood, thoughts, speech and action, the aim being to reduce stress on the patient. Improved behaviour should reduce stress on the carer and have benefits for professional health carers. Failing memory and diminishing cognitive skills are stressful but environmental factors may make things worse, and a quiet, well-heated, bright, unrestraining, calm environment may effectively improve behaviour in a disturbed patient. The creation of an appropriate environment should be encouraged by attending nurse and doctor.

Figure 10.2: Problem behaviour — a framework for action

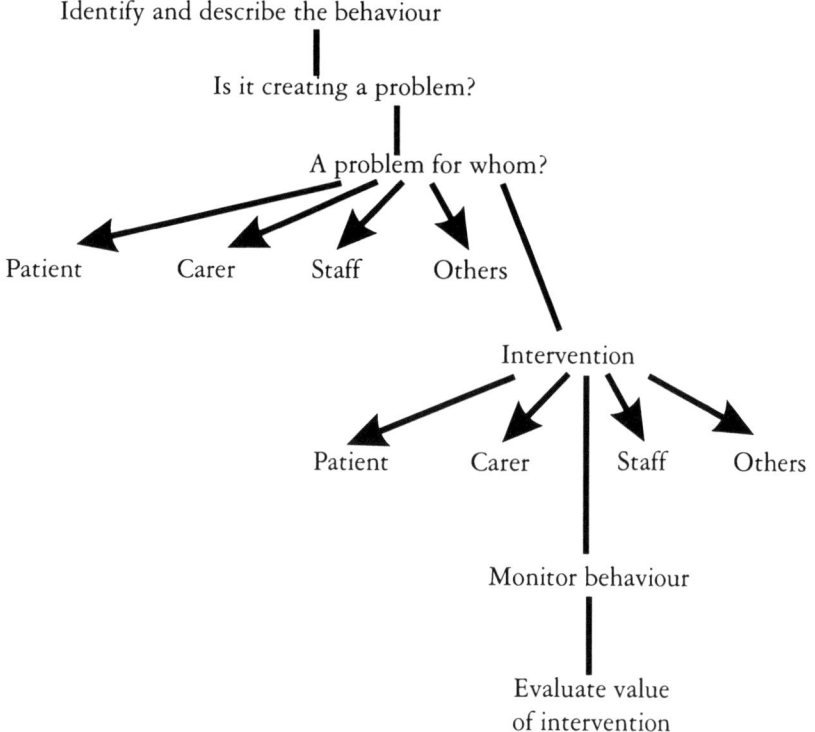

If the patient is cold, over-heated, incontinent, wet, hungry or in pain, he/she is likely to exhibit behavioural disturbance which needs to be addressed.

Disruptive behaviour can present as:
- wandering
- sundown syndrome
- aggression
- violence
- sexual exhibitionism
- over-reaction and catastrophic reaction.

In order to combat disruptive behaviour the problem has to be clearly defined and identifiable causes sought. Some can be eliminated and others ameliorated with appropriate action, followed by evaluation of the patient response to that action. A positive approach is to consider that difficult and antisocial behaviour is really a management problem which should prompt the following questions based on the problem-solving formula of what, where, when, and how?

A positive approach to behavioural problems

What exactly happens?

When does it occur?

How long does it take?

Where does it occur?

The doctor should remember that physical, auditory and sensory difficulties can cause external evidence of confusion and lead to disturbed behaviour, which may respond when functional problems are corrected. Decision-making revolves around prevention, amelioration, toleration and behaviour modification.

11
Caring for the carer

A 1993 survey by the Alzheimer's Disease Society found that about half of carers spent more than 80 hours per week caring for a relative or friend with the disease, 40% of carers had to access private savings, take out a loan or sell property to meet the financial demands of this care, and a remarkable 97% admitted to emotional problems varying from acute to chronic stress, tiredness, loneliness, isolation and depression. The majority of carers are close relatives, and a disproportionate number of them are female, and usually middle- or old-aged themselves. About one-third of carers have no other informal support. A quarter feel they are not coping and half of them find caring upsetting and the cause of practical problems which they find insoluble (Ford Valley Health Board, 1996). As about 80% of people with dementia are probably living within the community, frequently in their own homes, a large number of carers — usually women of late middle age — are affected in this care situation.

The NHS and Community Care Act, 1990 is likely to ensure that even more people with dementia will continue to live at home in the future. There are financial advantages to health and social services in keeping such people in the community. An hour's support care a week for a person in early stages of Alzheimer's disease may be sufficient to keep the individual out of hospital for a considerable length of time (Alzheimer's Disease Society, 1995). If the person with dementia lives alone the absence of this support will necessitate crisis intervention management by the GP and the health care team.

Considerable pressures are exerted on the physical and emotional reserves of carers, who may have to cope for 7–9 years with a deteriorating spouse or sibling. The need for care is constant and impacts very heavily on the carer's own life and quality of living (see Table 11.1). Some care problems are well tolerated and others, such as sleep disturbance by the patient are poorly tolerated (see Table 11.2). The common factor to most care problems is the demand on the care-givers' time. Carers become mentally exhausted, and can easily become isolated from society and suffer from what has been called *ongoing bereavement,* which occurs when the person is declining slowly from dementia. Grief is part of the bereavement process, but with a person undergoing the gradual loss of a loved one often associated with Alzheimer's-type dementia, there is no early relief from death. The burden is a continuing grief process which cannot be shared with the patient. Several other emotional problems arise in carers:

1. They may feel anger and aggression as a result of fatigue and frustration. Recent efforts in annual geriatric assessment have often left carers frustrated when the services that have been promised have never materialised.
2. They may feel guilty, possibly because they do not wish to carry the burden of care, or because they lose their temper with the individual concerned, or they wish to place the patient in respite care or short-term institutionalisation, or they absent themselves for short times from the caring situation.

Social isolation

Social isolation can occur when time demands on carers gradually force them out of leisure-time activities and social interactions away from the home. They curtail relationships and gradually focus all their activities on the patient and their environment, excluding conventional social support from friends, colleagues and associates which might help to diminish the personal stress that is inseparable from intimate dementia care.

Management of carers' problems

Respite interventions and individual psychosocial interventions are moderately effective in helping carers (Knight *et al*, 1993). The services most valued by carers are those which provide emotional support and practical help, rather than just respite care alone (Cunningham *et al*, 1995). Comprehensive support, including advice and information to individual carers and families, and the attendance at care-giver support groups reduces the need for spouses of patients with dementia to place husbands or wives in institutional care (Mittleman *et al*, 1993). The provision of written information about the illnesses and services, and practical advice on day-to-day management issues does appear to help reduce stress in carers (Toner, 1987).

The input of respite care and support services may help to alleviate anger at the burden imposed by the care situation.

Promises to provide additional services should only be made if they can be honoured and will be provided without a protracted delay. It is better not to make offers that are unlikely to materialise.

Guilt, anger and frustration may be worked out by careful counselling. Early diagnosis and telling the patient of the diagnosis may prevent the development of early guilt feelings and provide the opportunity for carry-over guilt, from earlier life events involving patient and carer, to be explored and discarded.

If these feelings are entrenched and do not respond to changes in the care situation or counselling, the possibility of carer abuse must be considered. Anger and frustration can precipitate physical and verbal abuse of the patient.

Financial support

Family carers sometimes have to be encouraged to seek financial support benefits to which the patient is entitled. The Attendance Allowances are awarded to those people needing constant care during the day or round the clock. They comprise:
- Disability Living Allowance (DLA) for those under 66 years
- Attendance Allowance for those aged 66 years or over.

The DLA has two elements: mobility and care. The latter is applicable to people with dementia and it is paid at three rates — the lower rate is suited to people in the early stages of the disease and the higher rate to those in the later stages.

Carers themselves who might otherwise have been working can claim Invalid Care Allowance. Age Concern produces a useful guide to welfare benefits called *Your Rights*. Carers should ensure that they receive the benefits to which they are entitled, which can be used to obtain the services of an occasional minder, sitter-in or home help to provide some respite from the unremitting demands of dementia care.

Table 11.1: Effects of care problems on the carer

	% reporting problem
Reduced social life	74%
Embarrassment	58%
Anxiety or depression	51%

Table 11.2: Patient behaviours that create problems for carers and are poorly tolerated by them

	% reporting problem
Dressing	69%
Washing	48%
Urinary incontinence	50%
Aggression	35%
Verbal abuse	27%
General wandering	30%
Faecal smearing	23%
Inappropriate urination	24%
Sleep disturbance	48%
Restless by day	52%
Cannot be left alone, even for 1 hour	68%

(Source: adapted from Gilleard, 1984)

Depression in carers

Studies have suggested that up to 14% of carers may suffer from clinical depression (Livingstone *et al*, 1996), with a third of them scoring high in terms of psychiatric disorder on the General Health Questionnaire. Depression is not an uncommon feature in carers who suffer from physical fatigue and often have interrupted sleep due to their patient's disturbed nocturnal activities. In general, the health of carers is poorer than that of control groups of non-caring subjects, and carers are more likely to have chronic illness.

Female carers are known to experience more nervous strain than male carers, with higher levels of depression and lower morale. This may be partly because male carers are much more likely to be offered formal support services than female carers. Many of these female carers are middle-aged, frequently daughters, and they usually have other roles with many varying responsibilities, including the care of their own children. Carers often feel that their role is unrecognised by society and by GPs in particular.

The effects of coping strategies

Carers who are able to maintain positive feelings towards their dementing relatives tend to have a lower level of perceived strain and a greater commitment to caring. Carers who followed an active management strategy with their charges, 'being firm in directing behaviour', have been shown to be significantly less likely to suffer depression than carers who did not. However, carers who prioritised their daily routines round the patient were more likely to be depressed. An active coping strategy of 'creating a larger sense of the illness' was associated with less depression (Saad, 1995). The type of coping strategy adopted by carers therefore appears to have an important relationship with depression Encouraging the right strategy in the carer may prevent the later onset of depression.

Poor previous familial relationships, where there was long-term hostility, make it unlikely that the carer will manage in the new dependent relationship. Much of the voluntary care is provided by middle-aged women who may themselves be failing physically, and may be incapable of carrying the burden without major community support. This may well be lacking if the pressure on them is not recognised.

Risk factors for depression

- Carers of elderly people with psychiatric disorders have an increased risk of depression.
- Depressive symptoms are more likely in women carers of people with dementia.

Case History

'One of my patients who had been a capable, caring mother and daughter until her 50s, gradually became worn down by the constant demands of the mother who developed dementia. Because the mother was living with the family, social workers were unprepared to put in any additional services. The lady was slow in applying for attendance allowance and felt it her duty to respond to her mother's needs rather than calling upon the state. However, in time her own health so deteriorated that she was forced to come to the surgery requesting help for her mother. After supporting the mother without state aid and recourse to any financial or resource input from the state for many years, in a time of need the social work department were unprepared to assess the mother for either respite or institutional care. In reaction to this response the carer's own health broke down and she developed recurrent chest infections and depression. The mother was admitted for short-term respite care but was referred on to long-term residential care where she died. The daughter was left feeling guilty that she had let her mother die in a "home". '

Caring for someone with dementia can stretch an individual's resources to the limit. The burden is far greater than the emotional one of caring for a physically disabled older person.

This burden largely relates to changes in the relationship with the dementia sufferer and the behavioural changes caused by the illness. These behavioural changes, associated with dis- inhibition, cognitive deficit and maladaptation, are difficult for the ordinary person to deal with. Failure to inhibit behavioural reactions, with resultant aggression, embarrassment and sexual misdemeanour, is difficult for family and carers to come to terms with.

It is believed that perhaps 18% of people with dementia are either verbally or physically aggressive to their carers, adding further to the stresses (Burns and Levy, 1993). Dyspraxia, self-care problems, loss of abilities to carry out activities of daily living, memory and learning problems, disorientation, wandering and personality changes are all distressing for close relatives. They can make life intolerable for the carer — especially when aggravated by night-time disturbance and wandering. Five factors have been identified as particular problem areas by Gilleard (1984):

1. Dependency — most carers complain that patients cannot be left alone, even for a short time (Askham and Thompson, 1990). They wander incessantly about the house, disrupting personal and social life and cannot be responsible for their own safety either within or outside the home environment.

2. Social disturbance — patients may disrupt conversations, disturb peace, and display inappropriate, socially unacceptable behaviour.

3. Coexisting physical disability engendered by their age and either not identified or ignored by family doctor.

4. Patients can make 24-hour-long demands.

5. Disorientation in time and place — patients may wander from home during the day or night through a period of 24 hours. There is no night-time respite for carers.

Support services

A wide range of formal support services are available from social work departments, local authorities and health services, including Meals on Wheels, mobile emergency care services, home helps and care attendants, laundry services, occupational therapy and the provision of respite and day care. These services enable carers to continue functioning and also improve the quality of life of the individual, but, they may not always offer the best response for individual patients or their carers.

Case history

'In this instance a 90-year-old female patient, almost totally isolated from the community due to deafness, major arthritic problems, incontinence and neuro-degenerative disease, is cared for by an 80-year-old sister who is blind and subject to fits. Twelve different carers organised by the social work department intervened on this patient's behalf between nine o'clock in the morning and nine at night. The carers vary in skills and interests, and there is no continuity of care, with the carers appearing one day and perhaps never again.'

This standard of care, although keeping the patient in the home environment, leaves much to be desired. However, Levin et al (1983) found that carers reported less stress when they were given greater formal support, even if they were not satisfied with the quantity and quality of services provided. Where respite programmes exist, carers also report improvements in their physical and mental wellbeing and an increase in their ability to continue care-giving support (Burdz and Eaton, 1988). There are several occasions when the stress felt by carers is particularly profound; one of these is when the initial diagnosis is made and carers want to know about the future effects of the disease and its prognosis. With the initial diagnosis there is often an unmet need for information for the family regarding the care situation they can expect to face in the future. At this time, relatives may deny the diagnosis or believe that the patient will respond differently from other sufferers whom they have known. They often feel anxious and frustrated.

Once the disease is well established, however, the carers often feel a sense of loss and ongoing bereavement. They feel that the person they once knew and lived with in close association for many years is already dead, although still physically present. Carers find withdrawn behaviour, when the demented person is silent and does not interact with family members, difficult to deal with. Exhibitions of unstable mood, where patients are angry, accusing and show big swings in emotions, also create difficult problems for carers. Home care, including nursing, medical and social input, appears to cost less than nursing home or hospital care, and is the current objective of Government policy (Figure 11.1). Nevertheless, carers/family carers pay an emotional price for this strategy and frequently suffer health problems in their endeavours to carry this particular burden.

Figure 11.1: The total cost of Alzheimer's disease in England 1990/1. Source: Gray and Fenn (1993)

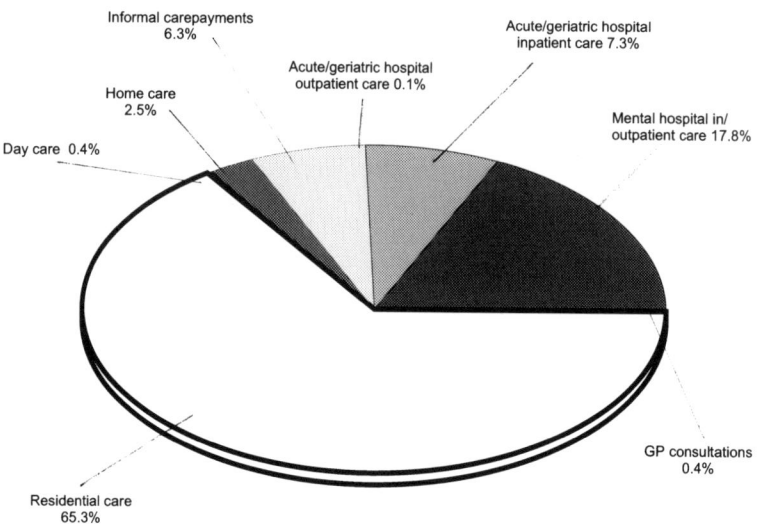

Reducing the stress in carers

Zarit, 1985, believes it is essential to give people accurate information about the disease and its progression in the family member. This helps to alleviate the sense of crisis brought on by the family's fears concerning the future progression of the disease. Lack of knowledge regarding what the carer should do or how to respond is highly stressful and providing adequate early information can put these problems into a workable perspective. Information need not necessarily come from the GP, but the GP should ensure that this is being provided by another health professional. The information can be both verbal and written but the health professional providing the information should first confirm that the carer does want the information about the disease process.

Information about available services does help to reduce stress. It is up to the health professional to organise support and be aware that failure to make such a provision after a promise to do so will lead to further frustration and added stress for the carer.

Half a million family carers are currently thought to be caring for someone with dementia, and in half of these cases the caring individual will be aged over 85 years (Cornwall, 1989). Although many female carers are older women, a considerable number are young and may have to give up jobs to care for their elderly relatives. This means a loss of income which is not made up by state benefits and allowances. They may lose out on pension contributions and on savings, a factor that is not always recognised by social or health authorities.

Early onset dementia

If the patient experiences an early onset dementia and has to give up a job because of the onset of the disease, with a resulting loss of two wage earners in the family, the financial, psychological and physical costs on the carer are compounded. Early onset dementia probably affects about 15 000 people in the UK (Jorm and Korten, 1988). State provision for these individuals and their carers is inadequate and placement into institutions is problematic and frequently inappropriate, creating an additional stress factor for family carers (Newens, 1994).

The mean age of carers is 66 years and over, with 40% of them reporting longstanding illness or disability. Two in three carers have lived with the person with dementia for more than 25 years (Levin, 1993). The stresses on carers are largely practical namely giving regular help with many aspects of personal care and dealing with incontinence, unsafe acts and wandering. There are often restrictions on carers' own leisure time and ability to leave home. The key worker, attending nurse or GP should be prepared to identify these concerns in an assessment process.

Once identified, it should be possible to ameliorate or eliminate the majority of stresses by practical input and external support services (Figure 11.2).

Figure 11.2: The service system response to the person with early onset dementia

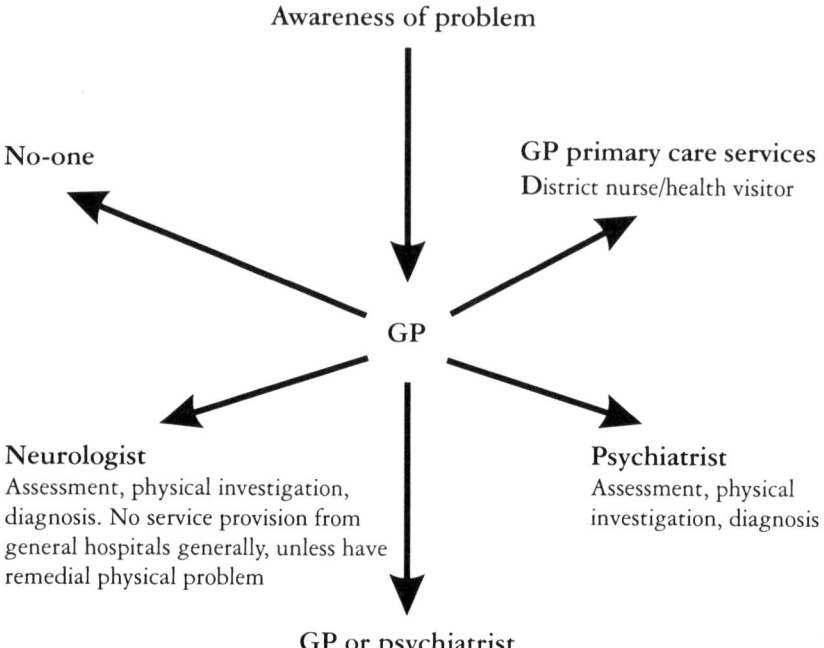

Respite care

Carers' needs and demands will depend upon the patient's stage of dementia. Respite care is very important to allow carers a break from tedious routine. It is known that half the carers never leave their relatives alone in the house, a third believe that they spend far too much time together with the patient, and the great majority believe that they are restricted from their own personal liberties by the caring process. Respite care will vary from area to area. Some of it can be voluntary body organised, through schemes such as Crossroads. Others may involve getting in care attendants. It behoves health professionals to ensure that the carer receives the Attendance Allowance and that this is utilised to engage a care attendant.

Respite care services in wards and day centres must also be utilised. It is best if this is done in anticipation of need, for waiting lists can be long. It is important that the GP involved in this process anticipates events, organises respite care dates and advises the carer of them in advance, so that he/she knows that the pressure will be relieved for a time-period in the near future. Packages of respite care are now legally required from health and social services acting jointly. They should be working in collaboration with the voluntary and private sectors to provide a comprehensive package of support. Giving intensive packages of respite care to the most severely dependent, behaviourally disturbed people is current governmental policy. This limits the scope, however, for using these services to prevent stresses on other carers, and for giving carers the opportunity to choose which respite services they would like.

Table 11.3: Needs and demands of people with dementia and their carers, at different stages of the disease

Early stages	
Carer's needs and demands	**Needs of people with dementia**
Information	Information
Counselling	Counselling
A social life	A social life

Middle stages	
Carer's needs and demands	**Needs of people with dementia**
Breaks	Familiar places
Normal social life	Familiar people
Shared care	Individual care
Peace of mind, rest	Taking risks/organised stimulation
Recognition	
Training	Lots of unconditional warmth
Someone to talk to	Someone to talk to
practical help	Others to take responsibility

End stages	
Carer's needs and demands	Needs of people with dementia
To relinquish all or much 24-hour care	Familiar places, familiar people
Counselling	Individual care
Self-esteem	Good physical care
	Psychological stimulation
	Environmental warmth

Source: Marshall M (1996) *'I can't place this place at all': Working With People With Dementia and Their Carers.* Venture Press, Birmingham.

Patient abuse

Family carers are often pushed to the limit of their endurance by the demands made upon them by the person with dementia. Exasperation, frustration, anger, social isolation, fatigue and exhaustion are unbearable associations in this caring situation. Carers can overreach their own physical and psychological capacity, and as many as 50% of all carers risk psychiatric illness (OPCS, 1988). There is a risk of overdependence on alcohol and drugs, and a further risk that they may begin to abuse their charges.

American studies have suggested that 2–10% of elderly people are at risk of abuse and a considerable proportion of these will be patients with dementia. Doctors report only 2% of all reports of suspected elder treatment which suggests a degree of under-reporting (Rosenblatt *et al*, 1996). This form of abuse does not seem to be related to social class or other social factors.

The majority of victims are female. A high proportion of spouse abuse involves women abusing husbands. When males are abusers, they are more likely to use physical force on the patient, whereas females tend to neglect their caring duties. Abuse can take several forms:

1. Psychological abuse, with embarrassment, humiliation and intimidation.
2. Physical assault with threatened and real assault taking place; physical assault can involve hitting and beating.

3. Neglect — the patient is deprived of heating, lighting and warmth.
4. Isolation — the patient is confined in a room, excluded access to public or family areas and denied social interaction.
5. Financial abuse — patients are persuaded to sign over authority to access their accounts or use their pension.
6. Over-sedation — with drugs, or failure to comply with provision of prescribed medication.
7. Physical restraint — the patient is confined by furniture or mechanical restraint to a small area.

When there are difficulties in communication abuse of people with dementia is not always easy to identify, but the attending GP should consider the possibility and pick up on pointers suggesting the absence of wellbeing. As a regular and impartial observer the GP should be sensitive to changes in the dynamics of the patient/carer relationship (Vernon, 1996).

Evidence of well being can be shown by:

1. Facial expression and countenance — does it indicate a good humour, enjoyment, distaste, fear?
2. Helpfulness — asked-for aid is proffered? Pleasure, facial expression and countenance and actions suggest enjoyment.
3. Affection — demonstrated by facial expression, non-verbal behaviour, gestures.
4. Emotional expression — a variety of responses given in appropriate ways.
5. Acceptance of others and willingness to participate in social events. Assertiveness, which is neither self-centred nor attention seeking.
6. Initiation of social contacts — without prompting.
7. Sensitivity to the needs of others. Patient is not stubborn or self-centred.

In the absence of many or all of these features the possibility of some form of abuse should be considered. Carers can either deliberately, or unintentionally, psychologically disturb patients. GPs should be aware of these possibilities and be prepared to discuss them with carers. More subtle forms of abuse are:

1. Infantilisation — the patient is treated like a baby.
2. Stigmatisation — the patient is referred to or labelled as mad, retarded or daft.
3. Invalidation — the patient's natural social interactions and comments are negated by the carer.
4. Objectivisation — the patient is treated like an object and kept clean and safe, but shown no respect as a human.
5. Intimidation — the patient may be verbally or physically abused or threatened by such abuse.
6. Disempowerment — the patient who could be involved in decision-making is refused the option of so doing.

All of these reactions diminish the patient's self-worth and status as an individual. Some professional carers can adopt similar attitudes and responses (Archibald *et al*, 1995). GPs should keep these reactions in mind and be prepared to intervene if they occur.

Some features of carer personality make abuse more likely. If an adult carer was abused as a child there is strong research evidence that he/she will act abusively in certain situations in adulthood. If the carer is making over-frequent visits to the GP, this may suggest that there are problems in the care situation. The majority of carers are highly committed, meet their responsibilities and perform a good job of caring for dementing patients. Some abuse results from the inadequacy of state support systems in meeting needs. Difficulty in access may be a sign of abuse when the individual restricts access to the patient or insists on being present during conversation with the patient.

Other factors which suggest that abuse may be likely, imminent, or exist are:

- expressive and receptive dysphasia in the patient
- recurrent reports of falls, minor injuries or burns
- evidence of neglect and malnutrition in the patient
- marked behaviour disorder, plus disinhibition or aggression in a patient
- refusal to allow patients into residential care.

Sexual abuse

Sexual abuse can also occur with these patients. Damage to frontal lobes of the brain in people with dementia can lead to disinhibition and the appearance of homosexual tendencies. Sexual advances made by these patients may meet with favour in some carers, and the patient may be subjected or submit to misuse and abuse (Archibald, 1994).

Management in cases of abuse

The early input of social health services can reduce pressure on the carer, and may reduce some of the frustrations and understandable feelings of aggression in carers. Referral to appropriate services may also bring respite and alleviate the carer from 24-hour attendance on the patient. The risk of financial abuse may be minimised if the financial situation is addressed early in the illness and appropriate protective measures introduced — an argument for early diagnosis (see Chapter 4). Drug mismanagement can be controlled by regular review of the medications and physical abuse should be picked up by regular examination of the patient (see Chapter 8). Abuse of the patient can be contained if it is identified. Identification requires its consideration by the care team in patient and carer contacts. Reducing the demands on the carer make it less likely that abuse will occur.

Refusal of services

The patient living alone and caring relatives frequently refuse to take up offered services. The isolated demented patient, who is unaware of the inadequacies of the home situation, may not recognise the need to enter a cared-for situation. Without recourse to compulsory procedures, which should be used only as a last course of action, one has to resort to encouragement and efforts to try to change such attitudes. An intervening bout of illness may be used as an opportunity to take up respite care. Hopefully, once the patient is exposed to the changed environment he/she may come to like it and be prepared to make the move.

Refusal by carers to allow patients to enter residential care does raise the possibility that some form of financial abuse is being perpetrated and there is financial advantage in keeping the patient at home. Carers often become over-committed to their charges and may need counselling and encouragement to accept proper care to safeguard their own health and wellbeing. Well-meaning, supportive interventions can be seen as intrusions by carers. They have to adapt to the idea of giving up care to an outside influence. Equally, institutional care is a very large intrusion, and is best approached by short weekly or fortnightly spells of respite care before longer-term commitment. Carers and families can be left with feelings of guilt about not coping well enough or not caring for long enough, and the GP should be prepared to explore these feelings and counsel the carer. Management in these situations is always one of compromise, agreeing to what patients and relatives find acceptable and weighing it against the risks to and best quality of life for the patient.

Care-giving families are often determined to continue caring even when formal support is not forthcoming (Levin et al, 1989). They often do so until a crisis point is reached, and this precipitates institutionalisation. Carers have been called the hidden victims of dementia, because in the caring process they have a price to pay in terms of physical health, emotional wellbeing, and social relationships (Zarit, 1985). Providing support for carers is a critical component of effective community-based dementia care and the GP must take the carer into consideration when dealing with this disease. Often their need for help at nights and week-ends is poorly addressed, and rarely met in full. Out-of-hours, in-home respite services have been poorly developed, although this is the service most sought after by carers. The GP should know where respite care may be obtained and should ensure that the facilities which exist in the neighbourhood are being tapped by this particular family unit. GPs have multiple roles to play in dementia management, but there is clear evidence that carers are still not satisfied with their involvement in professional support services (Brodaty et al, 1990). Carers care for many years without knowing about available support (Badger et al, 1990). The involvement of the GP and primary care team continues from diagnosis to the death of the patient and must include the carer (Briggs, 1993; Brodaty, 1990; Jacques, 1992).

Financial and legal concerns

Doctors are often asked for an opinion on a patient's mental capacity to make a decision; this is often a difficult problem to resolve (Arie, 1996). There is a risk of financial abuse when a person loses cognitive skills and cannot remember what has been done with money, how to access it, or even its purpose. One sound argument for making an early diagnosis of the condition is that it does permit the patient, in conjunction with the family, to make financial provisions to safeguard the future. A patient's pension from the Department of Social Services (DSS) can be signed for or collected by a patient's carer or other responsible person. If the patient goes into a nursing home setting, there are opportunities for misuse of these funds. There are instances where this money had been taken by the home without formal receipt and then a claim was made on death against the patient's estate for the same monies. While patients are mentally able, they can agree to arranging for someone else to handle their affairs. This agreement is called 'power of attorney'.

Power of attorney: This is drawn up by a lawyer and, once signed, remains valid as the person's illness progresses. It has to be done when the patient is still of sound mind and is restricted to financial matters. Once the patient becomes too confused, a power of attorney will not be granted. The legal arrangement then is for the court to appoint a 'curator bonis' to handle the person's money affairs. An *enduring power of attorney* continues in effect should the grantor become mentally incapacitated (England and Wales).

Curator bonis: In this instance, the sufferer does not have to give consent. The duty of the curator is primarily to preserve the estate of the client. The court usually appoints a lawyer or accountant as securitor, but it is an expensive process and is probably not worthwhile unless the estate is worth at least £50 000.

In some instances, especially when there has been abuse, there may need to be consideration of legal steps under 'guardianship' arrangements.

Guardianship

Guardianship under the UK Mental Health Acts safeguards patients with dementia. The procedure requires two independent medical opinions and the opinion of a mental health officer to confirm that an application is required.

Guardianship is intended to help people who have lost the ability to act in their own welfare interests. The guardian, when appointed, has the power to require the individual to attend for medical treatment, to live in a specified place, and to assist in providing access by doctors, mental health officers, or other specified persons. Guardians do not have any powers in relation to the patient's money or possessions, and they cannot consent to treatment on the patient's behalf. Social work departments often become involved in guardianship arrangements. A mental health officer (MHO) from the social work department will visit the patient and assess the need for guardianship. The MHO will then arrange for the patient's mental condition to be assessed by two doctors; if they support this application, it is submitted to the sheriff.

Tutor bond

Another alternative is a *tutor bond*. This is a person appointed by the court of sessions to take personal decisions on behalf of the mentally ill/incapable person. Tutors can also look after finances, and usually close relatives are appointed. This is an expensive procedure and is rarely used.

It is remarkable that one still meets carers who have not applied for the Disability Living Allowance (DLA) for those aged under 66 when they have been under financial duress. The money from these benefits can go towards buying in private home help or respite sitters to ease the burden on the formal carer. Despite intervention by health professionals, encouragement to apply for these benefits can be overlooked and some carers are very resistant to taking advantage of these state provisions. The attending doctor should confirm that applications have been made.

The patient's claims may be turned down. Re-application should be recommended for it invariably meets with success and makes some recompense to the carer who is trying to cope with the daunting demands of dementia. Many people with dementia are elderly, the last in a family line, and have outlived their associates. There is often no-one to act in their interest. Major decisions are made on their behalf by well-meaning health professional and social work interventionists. Many difficult fiscal, ethical and moral problems occur in their long-term management.

Advocacy

In some parts of the world such as Australia there is an advocacy service, where an individual or agency has a clear task of representing the interests of the person with dementia. Advocates are people with no vested interest, who represent the views of the people with dementia and the decisions that affect them. They are there to help work out what the person would have wanted to say and what decision might have been taken. They give the person with dementia a voice in a world where they are generally silent, and can assist in the decision-making progress at case conferences, offering a point of view from the patient's perspective. This service is poorly developed in the UK, but is a possibility that might be kept in mind by GPs involved in decision-making processes.

When advocacy should be considered (Burton et al, 1997):
- critical transitions, eg. when a patient is requiring admission to institutional care
- to resolve conflicts of interest between a patient and carer, such as during an assessment of needs
- with patients who lack family support and where the situation is deteriorating
- in case discussions where questions of risk are to be discussed
- where the patient's impairment causes communication difficulties.

In the early stages of illness it is appropriate for the doctor to suggest that the patient makes a will or ensures that a current one is up to date. Another consideration might be the creation of a *Trust*.

Trust

Money and property are handed over to trustees, with instructions for them to be used for the benefit of someone else, or to be handed over for the patient's benefit when the dementia worsens. If this is done it may avoid assessment by income support and DSS supplementation authorities, although it does count as capital when assessing the cost of local authority residential accommodation.

Compulsory removal from home

Few GPs enjoy making legal provisions for compulsory removal of patients from homes they have long occupied. There are often, however, considerable pressures placed on the GP by neighbours and other caring professionals, who insist that insanitary conditions, or other considerations, mean that the individual is not getting proper care and attention at home. The risk from hypothermia in unheated premises can be a real threat to life.

Compulsory removals can be instigated on the grounds of 'insanitary conditions' by a visiting regional medical officer, who is satisfied that removal is necessary and recommends to the council that this be done. The council then applies to the sheriff (procurator fiscal in Scotland) for an order. This procedure is very rarely used.

However, someone with moderate to severe dementia can be removed to and detained in a mental hospital under the Mental Health Acts. This can be done if:

- treatment in hospital is appropriate
- detention is necessary for the sufferer's health or safety or to protect other people.

This compulsory detention has to be authorised by the sheriff or relevant court officer after considering the medical reports of two doctors who have examined the sufferer. Detention orders last up to six months but may be renewed or terminated as necessary. The procedure which more frequently involves GPs is the order whereby a person can be detained without any court hearing for up to 72 hours, on the recommendation of single doctor and for a further 28 days if a psychiatrist advises that detention is necessary.

Most GPs try to avoid using compulsory powers to have their patients admitted. Most have had the sad experience of doing this and having the patient die within 24 hours, or having the patient returned to the community within 72 hours when there has not been support from the mental hospital for the patient to stay in hospital. Compulsory admission is always a very time-consuming task, invariably stressful and fraught with complications. The MHO from the social work department is normally involved, and the whole procedure usually arises from some urgent crisis intervention, a situation that is better pre-empted by anticipating care needs and making preparation for respite and hospital care as far in advance as possible.

Consent to treatment

An acute or chronic illness may make surgical or medical treatment necessary. In the case of a person with moderate to severe dementia, doctors can go ahead without consent if in their opinion proposed treatment is in the sufferer's best interests. GPs generally discuss proposed treatment with the person's close relatives or other carers to ascertain their views, but this arrangement is not binding on the doctor. Consent to treatment and research on people who no longer have the ability to understand the information provided in this regard is a controversial grey area. Mild dementia may not be incompatible with the ability to give informed consent. In determining **testamentary incapacity** the person should understand the nature of the act being undertaken. The existence of a degree of dementia does not preclude the making of an enduring power of attorney (Arie, 1996).

Advance statements/living wills

The concept of the production of a living will by a person when he/she is of sound mind and physically able to so do is now attracting attention. It offers people with dementia the possibility of influencing their terminal care at a time when they have lost the ability to voice their feelings about being allowed to die. In the absence of legalised euthanasia, these documents can have little impact on the death process. Such provisions, when made by people with dementia, complicate the terminal scene for the family doctor and are the probable source of many future courtroom battles. Considerable time is likely to pass before there are specific guidelines to guide the doctor through this medicolegal minefield.

The content of advance statements should include:
- a statement of the individual's preferences
- a statement of general beliefs and aspects of life
- the name of another person to be consulted, who will reflect the views of the patient, when a decision has to be made
- clear instruction refusing some or all medical procedures made by a competent adult which may have legal force
- a statement specifying the degree of irreversible deterioration after which no life sustaining treatment should be carried out.

Local authority and social work department obligations

The NHS and Community Care Act 1990 has introduced a further consideration in assessment, whereby carers have the right to be involved in the assessment of needs of the person for whom they are caring.

Local authorities have been advised that cognitively impaired people may require help from an independent person to represent their interest — an advocate. This form of representation has not yet been properly developed.

Conclusion

Dementia care has been associated with a high level of unmet need, mainly in terms of nursing, supervisory care and service provision. These demands, if not met by other service personnel, should be identified by the family doctor and every effort made to instigate the necessary support from caring agencies to fill the gap (Philip, 1989). Early diagnosis of the dementing process encourages involvement of the primary health care team, facilitates management before social crises occur and encourages remedial treatment and behaviour therapy that may be of benefit both to patient and carer (Copeland *et al*, 1986).

Misdiagnosis of the syndrome and associated depression, and failure to treat concomitant depression and physical illness in people with dementia, have been criticisms of family doctor care in the past. Hopefully, those who read this book will be encouraged to adopt the suggested guidelines and proposals for the management and care of these patients. Improved liaison and collaboration with the many health and social welfare agencies involved can only be to the advantage of those with this cognitively destructive, terminal illness and their family carers.

Appendix 1

Mini-Mental State Examination (MMSE)

Record response to each question

Orientation   Points

1. Year, month, day, date, season   /5
2. Country, county (district), town, hospital, ward   /5
   (room)

Registration

3. Examiner names three object (e.g. orange, ball,   /3
   key)

   Patient asked to repeat the three names and record them

   Score one for each correct answer

   Then ask patient to repeat the names three times to allow adequate learning for later recall purposes

Attention

4. Subtract 7 from 100, and 7 from the result etc.

   Stop after 5 (199, 93, 86, 79, 72, 65)

   Do not correct if errors made

   Alternatively spell WORLD backwards: DLROW
   Score the best performance on either task   /5

Appendix 1

Recall

5.	Ask for the names of the three objects learned earlier	/3

LANGUAGE   Points

6.	Name a pencil and a watch	/2
7.	Repeat, 'No ifs, ands or buts'	/1
8.	Give a three-stage command. Score one for each stage, eg.'take this piece of paper in your left hand, fold it in half, and place it on the ground'	/3
9.	Ask patient to read and obey a written command on a piece of paper, eg. 'close your eyes'	/1
10.	Ask patient to write a sentence. Score if sensible, eg. has a subject and a verb	/1

Copying

11.	Ask patient to copy intersecting pentagons	/1

Total score   /30

The test is said to be subject to variation based on cultural, educational and socioeconomic status:

    Standard cut-off: Normal = 24 or more
                                       Impaired = 23 or less

Age-related cut off: 40s normal = 29 or more

50s normal = 28 or more

60s normal = 28 or more

70s normal = 28 or more

80s normal = 26 or more

Less than 10 years of full time education: three extra errors allowed.

Doctors and nurses unfamiliar with use of MMSE should practice the procedure before commencing formal patient assessment with this measuring instrument (Folstein *et al*, 1995).

Appendix 2

Hachinski Ischaemic Score

A score of 4 or less is taken to be suggestive of Alzheimer's disease

A score of 7 or more suggests vascular dementia

Clinical date (history or clinical sign)	Ischaemic score
Abrupt onset	2
Fluctuating course	1
Nocturnal confusion	1
Relative perseveration of personality	1
Depression	1
Somatic complaints	1
Emotional incontinence	1
History of hypertension	1
History of strokes	2
Evidence of atherosclerosis	1
Focal neurological symptoms	2
Focal neurological signs	2
Stepwise deterioration	1

Hachinski, 1974

Appendix 3

Activities of daily living scale (Mahoney and Barthel, 1965)

Barthel index		Surname _____ Forename(s) _____ Sex _____ Address _____			
Date of examination		Before illness			
Bowels[1]	0 Incontinent 1 Occasional accident (once a week) 2 Continent				
Bladder[2]	0 Incontinent 1 Occasional accident (once per 24 hours) 2 Continent (for more than 7 days)				
Grooming[3]	0 Needs help with personal care 1 Independent (implements provided)				
Toilet use[4]	0 Dependent 1 Needs some help 2 Independent				
Feeding[5]	0 Unable 1 Needs help (cutting, spreading etc) 2 Independent (food within reach)				
Transfer[6]	0 Unable — no sitting balance 1 Major help (physical, 1 or 2 people) 2 Minor help (verbal or physical) 3 Independent				
Mobility[7]	0 Immobile 1 Wheelchair dependent 2 Walks with the help of one person 3 Independent				
Dressing[8]	0 Dependent 1 Needs help but can do half unaided 2 Independent (include buttons, zips, laces)				
Stairs[9]	0 Unable 1 Needs help (verbal or physical) 2 Independent up and down				
Bathing[10]	0 Dependent 1 Independent				
Total score (best = 20, worst = 0)					

Appendix 4

Over-75s assessment profile and check list (McIntosh, 1990)

Name	Name and relationship of caring relative or next of kin
Civil status M/S/W/D	Name ....
Date of birth	
Address	Address ....
....	....
Telephone	Telephone ....
Type of housing	

Services needed: R = required, P = provided, D = discontinued, Ref = refused					
Date of review					
Chiropody					
Day hospital					
Dental care					
Optician					
Audiometry					
District nurse					
Health visitor					
Social worker					
Home help					
Hospital					
Housing					
Medical emergency care service					
Meals on wheels					
Occupational therapists					
Others ( )					

Environment

Score	Household	Date				
0	Fully independent					
1	Friend or relative lives with them					
2	Friend or relative visits regularly					
3	Dependent on social services					
4	Dependent on local community nurses etc					
5	Combination					
	Sub-total					

Score	Bereavement of spouse or sibling					
0	None					
3	Less than 2 years					
5	Less than 6 months					
	Sub-total					

Score	Housing					
0	No problems					
1	Too big					
2	Too many stairs or similar					
4	Damp or in poor condition					
5	Multiple housing problems					
	Sub-total					

Score	Warmth					
0	Adequate					
3	Barely adequate					
5	Inadequate					
	Sub-total					

Appendix 4

Activities of daily living

Date

Score	Mobility					
0	Fully mobile					
2	Mobile with aids					
4	Housebound					
5	Bed or chairbound					
	Sub-total					

Score	Continence					
0	Fully continent					
2	Stress incontinence or urgency					
4	Day/night incontinence					
5	Incontinent of urine and faeces					
	Sub-total					

Score	Vision					
0	Satisfactory					
1	Uses vision aid					
3	Partially sighted					
5	Blind					
	Sub-total					

Score	Hearing					
0	No noticeable loss					
1	Satisfactory with hearing aid					
3	Unsatisfactory with/without aid					
5	Total deafness					
	Sub-total					

Activities of daily living

	Date					
Score	**Hygiene**					
0	Satisfactory					
1	Satisfactory with aids					
3	Bath or shower with assistance					
4	Dirty and unkempt					
	Sub-total					

Score	**Diet**					
0	Satisfactory					
1	Satisfactory with supplied meals					
3	Deficient					
	Sub-total					

Score	**Weight**					
0	Normal					
2	Moderately obese					
4	Underweight/obese					
5	Very underweight/very obese					
	Sub-total					

Score	**Sleep**					
0	Sleeps well without sedation					
2	Disturbed sleep					
3	Sleeps well with sedation					
	Sub-total					

Score	**Emotional assessment**					
0	No problems					
2	Discontented					
4	Very unhappy					
	Sub-total					

Appendix 4

Medication

	Date	Drug	Dose	Notes
1				
2				
3				

Medical assessment

Weight: BP:

Score 0 = no symptoms to 5 = severe symptoms at each assessment

	Date					
Cardiovascular						
Endocrine						
Gastrointestinal						
Genitourinary						
Locomotor						
Memory loss						
Nervous system						
Psychiatric						
Respiratory						
Skin						
Sub-total						

Score Totals

Medical					
Daily living					
Cumulative score					

At risk

H = high L = low M = medium

Received annual GP assessment (signature)

Refused offer of annual assessment

Developed by Iain B McIntosh

Appendix 5

Abbreviated Mental Test

- Age
- Time (to nearest hour)
- Address for recall at the end of the test, eg. 42 West Street. This should be repeated by the patient to ensure that it has been heard correctly.
- Year
- Name of hospital
- Recognition of two persons, eg. doctor, nurse
- Date of birth
- Year of First World War
- Name of present monarch
- Count backwards from 20

Each question scores one mark. Scores below 7 indicate the possibility of cognitive impairment

Hodkinson, 1972

Appendix 6

Geriatric depression scale (Sheikh and Yesavage, 1986)

The Geriatric Depression Scale (GDS) is a valid and reliable, brief rating scale that is useful for screening for depressive symptoms as well as for monitoring change. In less than five minutes it can be completed by an interviewer (or even be self-administered). It has been designed and validated for an elderly population since (unlike some other scales) it excludes somatic items which can be misleading because elderly people often have a variety of physical complaints.

Scoring the GDS

The elderly patient rings one response to each of the 15 questions.

All responses indicating depression are in bold on the example. The number of corresponding rings is totalled. A score of five or more indicates probable depression. 0–4 is normal.

Please answer all the following questions by ringing either 'Yes' or 'No'.

1.	Are you basically satisfied with your life?	Yes/**No**
2.	Have you dropped many of your activities and interests?	**Yes**/No
3.	Do you feel that your life is empty?	**Yes**/No
4.	Do you often get bored?	**Yes**/No
5.	Are you in good spirits most of the time?	Yes/**No**
6.	Are you afraid that something bad is going to happen to you?	**Yes**/No
7.	Do you feel happy most of the time?	Yes/**No**
8.	Do you feel helpless?	**Yes**/No
9.	Do you prefer to stay at home, rather than going out and doing new things?	**Yes**/No

10. Do you feel you have more problems with memory than most? **Yes**/No
11. Do you think it is wonderful to be alive now? Yes/**No**
12. Do you feel pretty worthless the way you are now? **Yes**/No
13. Do you feel full of energy? Yes/**No**
14. Do you feel that your situation is hopeless? **Yes**/No
15. Do you think that most people are better off than you are? **Yes**/No

References

Aarsland D, Cummings J, Kanfer D (1995) *Alzheimer's Re* 1(3): 133–6
Absher JR, Cummings JL (1994) Cognitive and non-cognitive aspects of dementia syndromes: an overview. In: Burns A, Levy R, eds. *Dementia*. Chapman & Hall, London: 59–76
Adshead F, Daycody D *et al* (1992) Brief assessment of dementia (BASDEC). *Br Med J* 305: 97
Alzheimer's Disease Society, England (1993) *Deprivation and Dementia*. DSDC, London
Alzheimer's Disease Society, England (1995) *Right from the Start*. ADS, London
Alzheimer's Disease Society (1995) *Dementia in the Community: Management Strategies for General Practice*. Alzheimer's Disease Society, London
Allan K (1994a) *Wandering*. DSDC, Stirling
Allan K (1994b) Dementia in acute wards. *Nurs Stand* 9: 11
Amar K, Wilcock G (1996) Vascular Dementia. *Br Med J* 312: 227–31
American Psychiatric Association (1994) *Diagnostic and Statistical Manual of Mental Disorders*, 4th edn. AMA, Washington DC
Anand R, Gharabami G, Enz A (1996) Efficacy and safety results of the early phase studies with escelon (ENA713) in Alzheimer's Disease — an overview. *J Drug Dev Clin Pract* 8: 1–14
Ancill RJ (1989) Cognitive-affective disorder — the co-presentation of depression and dementia in the elderly. *Psychiatr J Univ Ottawa* 14: 370–1
Ancill RJ (1993) Depression in Alzheimer's Disease. In Wilcock GK ed. *Management of Alzheimer's Disease*. Wrighton Biomedical Publications, Petersfield: 87–95
Anthony JC, Le Resche L, Niaz U *et al* (1982) Limits of the MMSE as a screening test for dementia and delirium among hospital patients. *Psychol Med* 12: 397–408
Archibald C (1990/1993) *Activities*. DSDC, Stirling
Archibald C (1994) *Sexuality and Dementia*. DSDC, Stirling
Archibald C (1996) Dementia: difficulties and dilemmas. *Psychiatry* 15: 19–21
Archibald C, Carver A (1994) *Food and Nutrition: Care of People with Dementia*. DSDC, Stirling
Archibald C, Chapman A, Weakes D (1995) *A Practice Guide for Community Nurses*. DSDC, Stirling
Argyll N, Jestice S, Brooke C (1985) The psychogeriatric patient: their supporters' problems. *Age Ageing* 14: 339–60
Arie J (1996) Some legal aspects of mental incapacity. *Br Med J* 313: 156–8

Armstrong-Esther C, Browne K (1986) Influence of elderly patient mental impairment on nurse patient interaction. *J Adv Nurs* **11**: 379-87

Askham J, Thompson C (1990) *Dementia and Home Care.* Age Concern, Institute of Gerontology, Research Paper 104

Badger F, Cameron E, Evers H (1990) Waiting to be served. *Health Serv* **15**: 54-5

Baldwin RC, Jollay DJ (1986) Prognosis of depression in old age. *Br J Psychiatry* **149**: 574-83

Barnes R, Veith R, Okimoto J et al (1982) Efficacy of anti-psychotic medication in behaviour disturbed, demented patients. *Am J Psychiatry* **139**: 1170-4

Bayer A, Woodhouse K (1993) *Care of the Elderly.* **4**: 36

Beck C, Medlin T, Hecthoff J et al (1992) Exercise as an intervention for behaviour problems. *Geriatr Nurs* September: 273-5

Berlinger W, Potter JF (1991) Lewy body index in demented out-patients. *J Am Geriatr Soc* **39**: 973-8

Blass J (1996) Age-associated memory impairment and AD. *J Am Geriatr Soc* **44**: 209-11

Blessed G, Tomlinson BE, Roth M (1968) Association between qualitative memory of dementia and of senile change in the cerebral grey matter of elderly subjects: Other factors in dementia. *Br J Psychiatry* **114**: 797-811

Bliwise DL (1994) What is sundowning? *J Aust Geriatr Soc* **42**: 1001-11

Bloom M (1993) Roles of GPs and other people in management of AD. In: Wilcock GK, ed. *Management of Alzheimer's Disease.* Wrighton Biomedical Publications, Petersfield: 59-76

Bowling A (1993) Nurse practitioners. *Practice Nurse* **6**(6): 508

Breteler M, Claus J (1992) Cardiovascular disease and distribution of cognitive function in elderly people: the Rotterdam study. *Br Med J* **308**: 1604-8

Breteler M, de Groot (1995) A prospective clinico-neuropathologic study of Parkinson's features in Alzheimer's disease. *Neurology* **45**: 1991-5

Briggs R (1993) The Marjorie Walker Lecture — What shall we do for dementia? *Geriatr Med* **23**: 41-5

Brodaty H et al (1988) Minimal brain damage in the adult. *Patient Management* August: 127-50

Brodaty H, Griffin D, Hadzi-Pavlovic D (1990) A survey of dementia carers. *Aust J Psychiatry* **24**: 362-70

Brodaty H, Howarth G, Mant A et al (1994) General practice dementia. *Med J Aust* **160**(3): 10-14

Brook P, Degun C, Mather M (1975) Reality orientation — a controlled study. *Br J Psychiatry* **127**: 42-5

Brooking (1980) Dementia and confusion in the elderly. In: Regen S, ed. *Nursing Elderly People.* Churchill Livingstone, Edinburgh

Brooks W, Whalley L (1992) *Prevalence of Dementia.* DSDC, Stirling

Bucht G, Sandman P (1990) Nutritional aspects of dementia. *Age Ageing* **19**: 532-6

References

Burdz M, Eaton W (1988) Effect of respite care on dementia and non-dementia patients and caregivers. *Psychol Ageing* 3: 38–42

Burns A, Hallewell C (1995) Old age psychiatry — 1995. *Update* 15 March: 341–7

Burns A, Levy R (1993) *Dementia*. Chapman & Hall, London

Burton A, Chapman A, Myers K (1997) *Dementia: A Practice Guide for Social Work Staff*. DSDC, Stirling

Butler R (1963) The Life Review: interpretation of reminiscence in the aged. *Psychology* 26: 65–76

Carr J, Marshall M (1993) Innovation in long stay care for people with dementia. *Gerontology* 3: 157–67

Chew CA, Wilkin D, Glendinning C (1994) Annual assessments of patients aged 75 years and over. *Br J Gen Pract* 44: 567–70

Clarke N, Jagger C, Anderson J *et al* (1991) The prevalence of dementia in a total population — a comparison of two screening instruments. *Age Ageing* 20: 396–403

Collinge J, Rossor M (1996) A new variant of Prion disease. *Lancet* 347: 916–7

Cooper B, Bickel H, Schaufele M (1992) The ability of the GP to detect dementia and cognitive impairment in elderly patients. *Int J Psychiatry* 7(8): 591–8

Copeland JRM, McWilliam MB, Davey BA (1986) Early diagnosis of dementia in the elderly. *Int J Psychol* 11: 63–70

Corder EH, Saunders AM, Stuttmatter WJ *et al* (1993) Gene dose of ApoE4 allele and risk of Alzheimer's disease in late onset families. *Science* 261: 921–3

Cornwall J (1989) *The Consumer's View*. Elderly People and Community Health Services, London: King's Foundation Centre

Cramond WA (1969) Organic psychosis. *Br Med J* iv: 497–500

Crook T, Bartus RT, Ferris SH *et al* (1986) AATU proposed diagnosis criteria and measures of clinical change. *Dev Neuropsychology* 32: 1569–73

Cunningham G, Dick S (1995) *'More than just a break'*. Action on Dementia, Scotland, Edinburgh

Davies M (1988) The role of GPs in supporting carers of the elderly in the community. *J R Coll Gen Pract* May: 194–5

Davis R (1989) *My Journey in Alzheimer's Disease*. Tyndale, Wheaton, Illinois

Dementia Services Development Centre (1995) *Social Work Departments*. DSDC, Stirling

Downs M (1994) *A Literature Review for the Northern Ireland Dementia Policy Scrutiny*. DSDC, Stirling

Edwardson I (1994)Lewy body dementia. *MRC News,* 64: 33–5

Elon M (1996) Geriatric medicine. *Br Med J* 312: 561–3

Farmer ME, White LR (1987) BP and cognitive performance. *Am J Epidemiol* 126: 1103–14

Feil N (1982) *Validation — The Feil Method*. Feil Productions, Cleveland, USA

Folstein MF, Folstein SE, McHugh PR (1975) Mini-mental status examination. *J Psychiatr Res* **12**: 189-98

Ford P, Heath H, eds. (1995) *Nursing Homes — Nursing values.* RCN, London

Forth Valley Health Board (1996) *Strategy for Services for People with Dementia.* Forth Valley Health Board, Stirling

Gale C, Martyn G (1996) Cognitive impairment and mortality in a cohort of elderly people. *Br Med J* **312**: 609-11

Gilhooley ML (1984) The impact of caregiving on carers. *Br J Med Psychol* **54**: 35-44

Gilhooley ML, Sweeting HR, Whittick J et al (1994) Family care of the dementing elderly. *Int Rev Psychiatry* **6**: 29-40

Gilleard C (1984) *Living with Dementia.* Croom Helm, London

Gilleard C (1997) Influence of emotional distress among supporters on the outcomes of psychogeriatric day care. *Br J Psychiatry* **150**: 219-23

Goldsmith M (1996) *Hearing the voice of people with dementia.* DSDC, Stirling

Goldwasser AM, Anerbach SM , Harkins S (1987) Cognitive affective and behavioural effects of reminiscence group therapy on demented elderly. *Int J Ageing Hum Dev* **22**: 209-22

Gordon D (1991) *Sampling Dementia Sufferers: Initial Experience in a Dundee Study.* Dept of Medicine, Ninewells Hospital, Dundee

Gordon DS, Gillies BA, McWilliam NG (1993) Spicker P.S. *Scott Med J*, **38**: 186-7

GrayFN(1993) *Alzheimer's Disease Media Pack.* Magellan Medical Communications Ltd, London

Green J, Timbury GA (1979) A psychogeriatric day hospital service. *Age Ageing* **8**: 49-53

Griffiths R (1988) *Community Care: Agenda for Action. A Report to the Secretary of State for Social Services.* HMSO , London

Gurland BJ, Copeland J, Kuriansky J et al (1983) *The mind and mood of ageing. Mental health problems of the community elderly in New York and London.* Croom Helm, London

Hachinski VC (1992) Preventable senility. *Lancet* **340**: 645-9

Hachinski VC, Lasson NA, Marshall J (1974) Multi-infarct dementia, a cause of mental deterioration in the elderly. *Lancet* **iii**: 207-9

Hanninen T, Hallikainen M, Hachinski VC et al (1995) A follow-up study of age-associated memory impairment. *J Am Geriatr Soc* **43**: 1007-15

Harvey R, Rossor M (1995) Treatment for Alzheimer's Type Dementia. *Practitioner* **239**: 440-43

Hodkinson HM (1972) Evaluation of mental test score for assessment of mental impairment in the elderly. *Age Ageing* **1**: 233

Holden N (1990) *Reality Orientation — Working with Dementia.* Winslow Press, Bicester

Holland AS (1994) Down's syndrome and dementia of Alzheimer's type. In: Burns A, Levy R, eds. *Dementia.* Chapman & Hall, London: 695-708

References

Horowitz A (1985) Family caregiving to frail elderly. In: Eisdorf C, ed. *Annual Review of Gerontology and Geriatrics*. JRS Springer Publishing, New York

House of Commons Social Services Committee (1990) *Community Care. 5th Report*. HMSO, London

Hunter DJ, Griffiths R (1988) *Community Care: Meeting the Challenge*. King's Fund Institute, London

Illiffe J (1992) What is the role of the GP? In: Bland R, ed. *Dementia and Assessment*. DSDC, Stirling

Iliffe J (1994) Targeting depression and dementia. *Geriatr Med* **24**: 55–57

Jacques A (1992) *Understanding Dementia*. Churchill Livingstone, Edinburgh

Janssen J, Gibberson D (1988) Remotivation therapy. *J Gerontol Nurs* **14** (6): 1–4

Jonker G, Launer L (1996) Memory complaints and memory impairment in older individuals. *J Am Geriatr Soc* **44**: 44–9

Jorm AF, Korten AS (1988) A method of calculating projected increase in numbers of dementia sufferers. *Aust NZ J Psychiatry*, **22**: 183–9

Jöst B, Grossberg G (1995) The natural history of Alzheimer's Disease — a brainbank study. *J Am Geriatr Soc* **43**: 1248–55

Katona K, Katona P (1996) A consensus opinion of depression in old age. *Geriatr Med* **26**: 45–7

Keady J (1996) Home alone — with dementia. *Practice Nurs* **7**(2): 3

Kellitt J (1989) Dementia and the elderly. *Br Med J* **9**: 34

Kelsey MC, Grossberg GT (1995) Serotonin specific re-uptake inhibitors and their role in weight loss. In: Vellas BJ, Jachet MD, eds. *Nutritional Intervention in the Elderly*. Springer Publishing Company, New York

Kendrick T, Burns T, Freeling D (1995) Randomised control of trial of teaching GPs to carry out structured assessments of their long-term mentally ill patients. *Br Med J* **311**: 93–8

Kennedy A, Rossor M (1993) Management of dementia — reasons for early diagnosis of dementia. *Practitioner* **237**: 103–7

Kist P, Hastie I (1995) Alzheimer's disease. *Postgrad Med J* April: 204–5

Kitwood T (1988) The contribution of psychology to the understanding of senile dementia. In: Geering B, Johnson M, Heller T, eds. *Mental Health Problems in Old Age*. Wiley, Chichester: 123–30

Kitwood T (1993) Towards a theory of dementia care — the interpersonal approach. *Age Society* **13**: 51–67

Kitwood T (1995) The technical, the personal and the framing of dementia. *Soc Behav* **3**: 161–79

Kitwood T, Bredin K (1992) *Person to Person. A Guide to the Care of Those with Failing Mental Powers*, 2nd edn. Gale Centre Publishers, Essex

Kivella SL, Pakhala K (1987) The progression of depression in old age. *Int J Geriatr Psychiatry* **1**: 119–34

Klerk RV (1994) How validation therapy is misunderstood. *J Dementia Care* **2**(2):14–16

Knapp MJ, Knopman DS, Solomon PR et al (1994) A 30-week randomised controlled trial of high dose tacrine in patients with Alzheimer's Disease. *JAMA* **271**: 985–91

Knight B, Lutzky S(1993) A metaanalytic review of interventions for caregiver distress. *Gerontologist* **35**: 240–8

Lai F, Williams R (1989) A prospective study of Alzheimer's disease in Down's syndrome. *Arch Neurol* **46**: 849–53

Larson EB, Kirkull WA, Bucher D et al (1987) Adverse drug reaction associated with global cognitive impairment in elderly persons. *Ann Int Med* **107**: 169–73

Lawlor BA, Aisen P, Green E et al (1997) Selegiline in treatment of behavioural disturbance in Alzheimer's Disease. *Int J Geriatr Psychiatry* **12**: 319–22

Lazarus LW, Newton M, Cohler B et al (1987) Frequency and prevalence of depression symptoms in patients with dementia. *Am J Psychiatry* **144**: 41–5

Ledesert B, Ritchie H (1994) Diagnosis and management of senile dementia in patients — arguments for standardisation of cognitive testing instruments. *Int J Geriatr Psychiatry* **9**: 43–6

Levin E, Sinclair I, Gorback P (1989) *Families, Services and Confusion in Old Age.* Avebury, Aldershot

Levin E, Sinclair I, Gorback P (1983) *The Supporters of Confused Elderly Persons at Home.* National Institute of Social Work, London

Levin E (1993) Care for the carers. In: Wilcock GK, ed. *Management of Alzheimer's Disease.* Wrighton Biomedical Publications, Petersfield: 211

Lewis C (1995) Living with dementia. *Psychiatry in Pract* **14**(2): 12

Liston EH (1978) Diagnosis delay in pre-senile dementia. *J Clin Psychiatry*, **39**: 599–603

Livingstone G, Mankela M, Katona L (1996) Depression and other psychiatric morbidity. *Br Med J* **312**: 153–6

McMichael S, Grice C, Gatwood F, McDowall S (1995) *Peacemaking between Tribes.* DSDC, Stirling

Maier S, Seligman M (1976) Dementia as a disability: learned helplessness. *J Exp Psychol* **103**(3): 46.

Mahoney F, Barthel D (1965) Fundamental evaluation. The Barthel Index. *Maryland Med J* February: 61–5

Malcolm D (1993) *Early Dementia and the GP.* DSDC, Stirling

Mann D (1995) How genetic causes of ATD further understanding of its pathogenesis. *Alzheimer Research* **1**(3): 119–21

Marshall M (1993) Wandering is a myth. *J Dementia Care* **1**(6): 14

Marshall M (1994) *'I can't place this place at all': Working with People with Dementia and their Carers.* Venture Press, Birmingham

Medical Research Council News (1994) *Uncovering the Seeds of Senile Dementia.* Medical Research Council News **64**: 29–32

Miller E, Morris K (1993) *The Psychology of Dementia.* Wiley Press, Chichester

Mittelman M, Ferris M, Steinbert C et al (1993) An intervention that delays

References

institutionalisation of AD patients. *Gerontologist* **33**: 730–40

Monteiro W (1995) *Change works. Neurolinguistic programming.* RLP Press, Bristol

Morris R, Baddeley A (1988) Primary and working memory in ATD. *J Clin Exp Neuropsychol* **10**: 279–96

Morton I, Bleathman C (1991) The effectiveness of validation therapy in dementia — a pilot study. *Int J Geriatr Psychiatry* **6**(15): 327–30

Murphy C (1994) *It Started with a Sea-shell.* DSDC, Stirling

McGrath A, Jackson G (1996) Survey of neuroleptic prescribing in residents in nursing homes in Glasgow. *Br Med J* **312**: 611–12

McIntosh I (1988) Geriatric surveillance and management using a 2-year trained nurse. *Scott Medicine* **5**: 332–3

McIntosh I (1990) A ready made package for screening the over-75's. *Geriatr Med* **20** (1): 1–5

McIntosh I (1993) Should we screen the elderly? *Med Monitor* 2 June: 32

McIntosh I (1996) Declining care with advancing years. *Scott Medicine* **15** (4): 3

McIntosh I (1997) Annual Geriatric Surveillance and Assessment. In: Beales D, Denholm M, Tulloch eds. *Community Care of Older People.* Radcliffe Press, Abingdon, Oxon

McIntosh I, Power K (1993) Elderly people's views of an annual screening assessment. *J R Coll Gen Pract*, **43**(370): 189–93

McIntosh I, Power K (1994) A price to pay for screening the elderly. *Geriatr Med* **24**: 11–12

McIntosh I, Swanson U, Power K et al (1997) GP stress and dementia management. *Scott Med* **16**: 7–8

McIntosh I, Woodall K (1995) *Dementia Management for Nurses and Community Care Workers.* Quay Books, Mark Allen Publishing Group, Dinton, Salisbury

McIntosh I, Young M, Stewart T (1988) A GP Geriatric Surveillance Scheme. *Scott Med J* **33**: 332–3

McKhann G, Drachmand D, Folstein M (1984) Clinical Diagnosis of Alzheimer's Disease. *Neurology* **34**: 939–944

McKeith IG, Fairbairn AF, Bothwell RA (1994) An evaluation of predictive value and interrated reliability of clinical diagnosis criteria for senile dementia of Lewy body type. *Neurology* **44**(5): 872–7

McLean S (1987) Assessing dementia, Part 1 — Difficulties, definition and diagnosis. *Aust NZ J Psychiatry* **21**: 142–74

McLean S (1993) Practical management of Alzheimer's disease. *Mod Med Aust* April: 16–87

MacLennan J, Murdoch P, McIntosh I (1993) *Dementia Touches Everyone — A Training Guide for GP Trainers and Registrars.* DSDC, Stirling

McMurdo ET, Thompson P (1997) How memory clinics can help primary care. *Scott Medicine* **16**: 9

McShane R, Hope T, Wilkinson J (1994) Tracking patients who wander. *Lancet* **343**: 1274

McShane R, Keene J, Gedling K *et al* (1997) Do neuroleptic drugs hasten cognitive decline in dementia? *Br Med J* **314**: 266-70

McWhirter M (1987) A dispersed alarm system for the elderly. *J R Coll Gen Pract* **37**: 244-7

Navia BA (1994) Dementia. In: Burns A, Levy R, eds. *AIDS*. Chapman & Hall, London: 763-80

Newens A, Forster DP, Kay D (1994) Referral patterns and diagnosis in pre-senile dementia implications for GPs. *Br J Gen Pract* **44**: 405-7

Neutel C, Hirdes J, Maxwell C *et al* (1996) New evidence on benzodiazepine use and falls. *Age Ageing* **25**: 273-8

National Health Service Medical Economics (1993) *New World, New Opportunities*. HMSO, London

North England Evidence Based Guideline Project (1997) *Primary Care Management of Dementia*. Department of Primary Care, University of Newcastle upon Tyne

O'Connor DW, Pollitt PA, Hyde JB *et al* (1988) Do GPs miss dementia in elderly patients? *Br Med J* **297**: 1107-40.

O'Connor DW (1993) Early intervention in dementia. *Br Med J* **301**: 871

O'Hanlon JD (1996) Antidepressant therapy and behavioural competence. *Br J Geriatr Pract* **50**: 381-88

O'Hanlon P (1987) Team approach soothes GP fears and improves service. *Geriatr Med* **17**: 43-6

Olley P (1996) Declining care with advancing years. *Scott Medicine* **15**(4): 5

O'Neill DD, Surmon DJ, Wilcock GK (1992) Longitudinal diagnosis of mental disorders. *Age Ageing* **21**: 393-7

Ohkura T (1995) Long-term oestrogen replacement therapy in female patients with dementia of Alzheimer's type. *Dementia* **6**: 99-107

Ott A, Breteler M (1995) Prevalence of Alzheimer's Disease and vascular dementias; association with education. *Br Med J* **310**: 970-3

Philips JM (1992) Geriatric planning. *World Hospitals* **28**: 117

Philp I, Young J (1988) Audit of support given to lay carers of the demented elderly. *Health Bulletin* **46**: 93-7

Philp I (1989) Challenge of dementia to GPs. Five areas of attack. *Geriatr Med* **19**: 19-28

Philip I (1995) *Practice Guide for Community Nursing*. DSDC, Stirling

Poirier J, Davignon J, O'Connor DW *et al* (1993) Apolipoprotein E polymorphism and Alzheimer's disease. *Lancet* **342**: 679-9

Pollitt PA, Anderson I, O'Connor DW (1991) For better or worse — the experience of caring for an elderly dementing spouse. *Ageing Soc* **11**: 443-69

Post SG, Whitehouse PJ (1995) Fairhill Guidelines on ethics of care with people with Alzheimer's disease. *J Am Geriatr Soc* **43**: 1423-9

Rabins PV, Mace NL (1986) Some ethical issues in dementia care. *Clin*

References

Gerontologist **5**: 501-12

Rabins PV, Nicholson MC (1991) Acute psychiatric hospitalisation for patients with irreversible dementia. *Int J Geriatr Psychiatry* **6**: 209-11

Rapp M, Flint A *et al* (1992) Behaviour disturbance in demented elderly. *Can J Psychiatry* **37**: 251-7

Rawlinson A, Brown A (1993) The community psychiatric nurse. *Scott Medicine*, **11**(6): 8-9

Reisberg B (1988) Functional assessment staging (FAST). *Psycho- Pharmacol Bull*: 653-9

Renvall M, Audrey A (1993) Body composition of patients with Alzheimer's disease. *J Am Diet Assoc* **93**: 47-52

Richards M, Reade T, Peart J *et al* (1996) Antithrombotic medication may protect cognitive function in old people at risk from cardiovascular disease. *Lancet* Conference: 'The Challenge of Dementia, 1996', Edinburgh

Ritter L (1991) Developing a therapeutic activities programme. In: Sloane P ed. *Dementia Units in Long-Term Care*. J Hopkins University Press, Baltimore

Rogers SL Friedhaft LT (1996) The efficacy and safety of donepezil in patients with Alzheimer's Disease. *Dementia* **7**: 293-303

Rosenblatt D, Kwung-Hwan Cho (1996)Dementia Care. *J Am Geriatr Soc* **44**: 65-70

Rossor M, Iverson LL, Reynolds GA *et al* (1984) Neurochemical characteristics of early and late onset types of Alzheimer's disease. *Br Med J*, **288**: 961-4

Rossor M (1993) Alzheimer's disease. *Br Med J* **307**: 779-82

Rossor M (1994) Uncovering the seeds of senile dementia. *MRC News* **64**: 29-32

Roth A, Fonagy P (1996) *What works for whom. A critical review of psychotherapy research*. Guildford Press, England

Rovner B, Steel C (1996) A randomised trial of dementia care in nursing homes. *J Am Geriatr Soc*, **44**: 7-13

Royal College of Nursing (1993) *The Value and Skills of Nurses Working with Older People*. RCN, London

Royal College of Nursing (1994) *Guidelines for Assessing Mental Health Needs in Old Age*. RCN, London

Royal College of Nursing (1991) *Older People and Continuing Care*. RCN, London

Rozzini R, Ferrucci L, Losonczy K *et al* (1996) Protective effect of chronic NSAID use on cognitive decline in older persons. *J Am Geriatr Soc* **44**: 1025-29

Rubinsztein DC (1995) Dementia assessment. *Psychol Med* **25**: 223-9

Saad K, Hartman Ballard M (1995) Coping by the carers of dementia sufferers. *Age Ageing* **24**: 495-8

Saletu B, Möller HJ, Grünberger J *et al* (1991) Propentofylline in adult onset cognitive disorders. *Neuropsychobiology* **24**: 173-84

Salzman C (1990) Practical considerations in the pharmacological treatment of

depression and anxiety in the elderly. *J Clin Psychol* 51(1): 40-3
Schoenberg B, Kakman, Okazati H (1987) Alzheimer's disease and dementing illness in a US population. *Ann Neurol* 22: 724-9
Schneider LS, Pollock VE, Lyness SA (1990) A metaanalysis of controlled trials of neuroleptic treatment in Dementia. *J Am Geriatr Soc* 38: 553-63
Secretaries of State for Health and Social Security (1989) *Caring for People*. HMSO, London
Senna TP, Palla K (1994) Effect of Omnibus Reconciliation Act on antipsychotic prescribing in nursing homes. *J Am Geriatr Soc* 42: 648-52
Sheikh JA, Yesavage JA (1986) Geriatric Depression Scale (GDS). In: Brink T ed. *Clinical Gerontology: A Guide to Assessment and Intervention*. Howarth Press, New York
Shua-haim JR, Gross JS (1996) Alzheimer's syndrome NOT Alzheimer's disease. *J Am Geriatr Soc* 44: 96-7
Scottish Intercollegiate Guidelines Network (1997) *Interventions in the management of behavioural and psychological aspects of dementia*. SIGN, Edinburgh
Skoog I, Leunfelt B, Landahl S *et al* (1996) Fifteen year longitudinal study of blood pressure study and dementia. *Lancet* 347: 1141-5
Smith R (1995) Proposals on poorly performing drugs. *Br Med J* 311: 402
Somerfield MR, Weisman CS, Ury W *et al* (1991) Physician practice in diagnosis of dementing disorder. *J Am Geriatr Soc* 39: 172-5
Scottish Health Purchasing Information Centre (1997) *Report on Dementia*. SHPIC, Edinburgh
Stilwell B (1982) The nurse practitioner at work. *Nurs Times* 78(43): 1799-1803
Stuss BT, Metran N, Guzman A *et al* (1996) Do long tests yield a more accurate diagnosis of dementia than short tests? *Arch Neurol* 53: 1033-9
Sutcliffe D (1990) Alzheimer's disease. Why the GP may not seem to care. *Horizon* May: 273-4
Takashi A, Tetsuhiko K (1996) Predictors of fall related injury in elderly people with dementia. *Age Ageing* 25: 22-8
Tand M, Jacobs D (1996) Effects of oestrogen during the menopause on risk and age at onset of AD. *Lancet* 348: 429-32
Thompson TL, Filley CM, Mitchell WD (1990) Lack of efficacy of hydrazine in patients with Alzheimer's disease. *N Eng J Med* 323: 445-8
Tinetti M, Doucette J, Claus E, Marotto R (1995) Risk factors for serious injury during falls by older people in the community. *J Am Geriatr Soc* 43: 1214-21
Tobianski R (1993) Understanding dementia. *J Dementia Care* 1(1): 26-9
Tombaugh TN, McIntyre NJ (1992) MMSE — a comprehensive review. *J Am Geriatr Soc*, 40: 923-35
Tomlinson B, Blessed G, Roth M (1970) Observations on the brains of demented old people. *J Neurological Science* 7:205, 242
Toner HL (1987) Effectiveness of a written guide for carers of dementia sufferers. *Br J Clin Soc Psychiatry* 5: 24-6

References

Tooth J (1995)Design for Living. *Scott Medicine* **15**: 12–13
Twigg J (ed) (1992) *Carers, Research & Practice*. HMSO, London
Vernon MJ (1996) Elder abuse. *Geriatr Med* **26**(1): 21
Victor M, Adams R , Collins G (1989) *The Werniche-Korsakoff Syndrome in Related Neurological Disorders* (2nd edn). FA Davies, USA
Watkins M (1988) Lifting the Burden. *Geriatr Nurs Home Care* October: 17–19
Watkins PB, Hyman J, Zimmerman MD et al (1994) Hepatotoxic effects of tacrine administration in patients with Alzheimer's Disease. *JAMA* **271**: 982–8
Wilcock GK ed. (1993) *Management of AD*. Wrighton Biomedical Publishing, Petersfield
Wilcock G (1994) Tacrine for Alzheimer's disease. *Age Ageing* **23**: 353–5
Wilcock GK, Ashworth DL, Langfield JA, Smith PM (1994) Detecting patients with ATD suitable for drug therapy: comparison of the methods of assessment. *Br J Clin Pract* **44**: 30–3
Wilkieson C, Campbell A, McWhirter M et al (1996) Standardisation of health assessments for patients aged 75 years and over. *Br J Clin Pract* **46**: 307–8
Will RG, Ironside JW, Couseus SR et al (1996) A New Variant of Creudzfeldt Jacob Disease in the UK. *Lancet* **347**: 921–5
Wilson RS, Evans D (1996) How clearly do we see memories? *J Am Geriatr Soc* **44**: 93–4
World Health Organization (1993) *ICD-10 Classification of Mental and Behavioural Disorders*. WHO, Geneva
Yesavage J, Brink T (1983) Development and validation of a geriatric depression scale. *J Psychiatr Res* **17**: 37–49
Young M, Chamoue A (1989) Evaluation of Elderly Screening. *Scott Medicine* **5**: 10–11
Zarit SH, Orr NK, Zarit JM (1985) *The Hidden Nature of AD: Families Under Stress*. University Press, New York
Zgola J (1990) Therapeutic activities. In: Mace AM, ed . *Dementia Care – Patient, Family and Community*. John Hopkins University Press, London

The Dementia Services Development Centre wishes to thank the Medical Insurance Agency for financial assistance with this project.

Index

A

The Alzheimer's Disease Society 3
abbreviated memory test 63
abbreviated mental test vi, 35, 84
ABC technique 123
abnormal cerebral circulation 57
acetylcholine 13, 17, 20, 94, 97
acetylcholine esterase inhibitors vi, 95
Activites of daily living: Barthel Index vi
activities in daily living 23
activities of daily living 21, 24, 37, 52, 88
activity programmes 80, 116
acute confusion 133
advance statements/living wills 157
advising the patient 30
  catastrophic reaction 30
advocacy 154
advocate 158
aetiology of attend 11
age-associated memory impairment 49
aggression 24, 59, 124, 135, 139, 142
  coping with 125
agitation 123
agnosia 25-6
AIDS related dementia 18
akathisia 103
alcohol 39
alcohol abuse 43
alcoholism 65
  chronic 42
aluminium 11

Alzheimer's disease 14, 40, 42, 44, 49, 51, 55
  early onset 53
  late onset 53
Alzheimer's disease assessment scale — cognitive subscale (ADAS-COG) 99
Alzheimer's Disease Society 7
Alzheimer's Disease Society, 1995 4
Alzheimer's-type dementia 9, 12, 28, 44-5
  advising person of diagnosis 29
  disease duration 8
amnesia 25-6
AMT 38, 60
amyloid 94-5
amyloid precursor protein 66-7, 94
anaemia 42, 79, 133
annual geriatric assessment 63, 82, 87
annual geriatric assessment programme 70
annual geriatric screening 36
annual geriatric surveillance 86
anticholinesterases 94
antidepressants 42
antipsychotics 102
anxiety 24, 47, 50, 139
anxiety disorders 107
anxiolytics 106
aphasia 25-6, 52
apo E13, 416
apolipoprotein E 96, 445
apolipoprotein E 445
apoliproteins 13
APP 12, 95
apraxia 25-6
arteriosclerosis 16
arteriosclerotic disease 42
aspirin 108

184

Index

assessment
  global approach to 73
assessment procedures v, 36
assessment programmes 36
assessment protocol 37–8
atherosclerosis 119
atropine psychosis 103
Attendance Allowance 138, 146
autopsy 27

B

Barthel Activities of Daily Living Index 84
BASDEC 60
behaviour disorder 150
behavioural changes v, 24
  aggression 25
  disinhibition 25
  disorientation 25
  self-neglect 25
  sundowning 25
behavioural disorders 102
behavioural disturbance 80, 104
behavioural management techniques 133
behavioural problems 40, 72, 102, 122
benign senile forgetfulness 49
beta-amyloid 10, 13
beta-amyloid protein 12
beta-blockers 106
Binswanger's disease 15
bizarre behaviour 48
blood coagulation 64
blood investigation 62
blood investigations 42, 64, 66
bovine spongiform encephalopathy 19
brain biopsy 42
brain deficits 22
brief assessment of depression schedule 35

C

The Community Care Act 1990 75

carbamazepine 106
cardiovascular system 64
care 2
  shortfall 2
care attendants 90
care givers 118
care management
  psychological methods of 114
care models 84, 93
care team 45
carer 8, 28
  caring for vi, 136
  stress 8, 32, 72
carer support 92
carotid stenosis 108
catastrophic reaction 23, 120, 135
causes of dementia v, 17
  vitamin deficiencies 17
cerebral hemispheres 10
cerebral infections 14
cerebral softening 16
cerebrovascular disease 14
cerebrum 16, 20
chest X-ray 44
chlormethiazole 105–6
choline esterase inhibitors 94
chromosome 14 12, 67
chromosome 19 12
chromosome 21 12, 18, 66, 95
  mutations 12
classification of dementia 21
clinical presentation v, 22
  denial 23
clinical psychologist 47
clinical social worker 48
cognition 24, 26, 52
cognitive ability
  objective assessment 41
cognitive assessment 38
cognitive changes v, 24
cognitive decline 34, 119
cognitive deficiencies 119
cognitive deficiency and

behavioural problems vi
cognitive function 34, 65, 76
cognitive performance 76
cognitive screening test 38
cognitive testing 58
cognitive testing scale 59
cognitive tests 34, 63
cognitively impaired 29
communication 110-1
  barriers to good communication 111-12
  non-verbal input 113
  verbal input 112
communication problems 113
community care
  key components 91
Community Care Act, 1991 7
Community Care Act, 1990 89
community dementia teams 88
community dietician 88
community mental health teams 92
community nurses 63
compulsory removal 155
computed tomography 62
computerised tomographic scanning 20
computerised tomography 44, 60
conclusion vi
confusion 43-4, 50, 53, 60, 105
  acute 56
confusional states 40, 42, 54-5, 62, 72, 107
consent to treatment 156
coping strategies 140
Creutzfeldt-Jakob disease 19
CT 46-7
CT brain scans 64
curator bonis 74, 153

D

the differential diagnosis v
day care 92
defects in neurotransmitter 19
delirium 56, 61, 63, 107

delusional ideas 40
delusions 24, 52, 54, 102, 107, 119
dementia 3, 8, 61, 63
  definition 6
  diagnosis of 28
  holistic approach 82
  syndrome 6-7
  presentation 6
  prevalence of 7-8
dementia — the syndrome v
  definition v
  size of the problem v
dementia care
  multidisciplinary involvement in 71
dementia care mapping 80
dementia management
  non-drug interventions 110
dementia stress management model 85
dementias
  vascular-induced 62
demographic trends 8
depression vi, 23-4, 30, 33, 39, 42, 47, 50-66, 79-80, 100, 106, 123, 130, 139, 141
  underdiagnosed 57
depression and dementia v
depression assessment scale 59
depression rating scales 62
depressive illness 33
  misdiagnosed 68
detection and early diagnosis v
detection rate for dementia 34
diabetes 64, 108
diagnosis 1, 39, 41, 46
diagnosis of dementia 6
differential diagnosis 50
Disability Living Allowance 138, 154
disempowerment 150
disinhibited 54
disinhibition 24, 25, 102, 119-22, 132, 141, 150-1

Index

disorientation 24, 142
disturbed behaviour 40, 102, 110
disturbed sleep 128
Donepezil (Aricept) 99
Down's syndrome 12, 18, 66
drop-in centres 92
drug management 94
drug management of dementias and behaviour problems vi
drug medication 42, 80
drug research approaches to ATD vi
drug therapy for sleep disturbance vi
drug treatment for depression vi, 100
DSM-IV criteria for diagnosis of Alzheimer's disease v
dysphasia 150
dystonic reactions 103

E

early diagnosis 28, 31, 33, 153
early onset dementia 8, 145–6
ECG 47
EEG 47
Elderly Assessment Profile and Checklist 84
electroencephalogram 60, 62
emotional changes v, 24
encephalitis 18
endocrine disorders 18
endocrine disturbances 57
erythrocyte sedimentation rate (ESR)43
Exelon 99
expressive therapies 116
expressive therapy 83

F

faecal incontinence 130
falls 53, 133, 150
familial ATD 12
    early onset 12
    genetic causes 12
    late onset 12

family carers 115–16, 130,143,145
financial abuse 149–52
financial and legal concerns vi
fits 23
fluoxetine 101
focal neurological deficit 65
folic acid 17
forward planning 32
frontal lobe tumours 54
full blood count 43
functional deficits 22

G

the GP's role in management v
gatekeeping 90
GDS 60
genetic testing 45
geriatric annual surveillance 87
geriatric assessment 38
geriatric assessment protocol 41
geriatric depression scale vi, 35, 84
geriatrician 47
glial activation limiter 97
glucose 43
GPs 1, 2, 28, 30–6, 45, 47, 50, 63, 70, 78, 89
    family doctors 4
    GP's sole responsibility 5
    GPs' roles 36, 68, 152
GP's role in management 69
guardianship 74, 153
guidelines 73
guidelines for assessing mental health needs in old age 83
guidelines for good practice v, 72

H

a holistic view 27
Hachinski ischaemic rating scale 62
Hachinski Ischaemic Score vi, 84
hallucinations 24, 39, 53–6, 59, 102, 107, 122
haloperidol 103
Hamilton depression 60
head injuries 18, 39

health link workers 87
health visitor 38, 63, 87
hearing loss 75
hepatic disease 42
hippocampal damage 10
history from the carer 40
history taking 39
HIV infection 18
holistic approach 85
holistic care 87
home care service 91
home helps 90
hormone replacement therapy 96
Huntington's disease 14
hypercholesterolaemia 108
hyperparathyroidism 43
hypertension 17, 42, 53, 64, 108
hypnotics 106
hypothyroidism 54–5, 66
hypoxia 57

I

impaired memory 58
incontinence 23, 75, 105, 121,130, 145
infantilisation 149
infarcts 44
infection 42, 57
infections 18
inflammatory 19
inflammatory systemic disease 14
intervention programme 68
intimidation 150
intoxication 56
intracerebral lesions 57
Invalid Care Allowance 138
invalidation 150

K

Korsakoff's syndrome 20, 65
   confusion 65
   memory loss 66

L

language disorders 24
Lewy bodies 16–17

Lewy body type dementia 14, 16, 42, 50–5, 94, 103, 106
life book 118
life review 88
life reviews 83
lithium 106
liver function tests 43
lofepramine 101
long tract signs 17
long-stay placement 46

M

a multidisciplinary approach 28, 154
magnetic resonance imaging 44
magnetic resonance imaging (MRI) scan 35
making the diagnosis v
   advantages to patient, carer and doctor v
malnutrition 42, 44, 57, 75, 88,150
management 3
   nihilistic 36
management of carers' problems 137
management of challenging behaviour vi
management of urinary incontinence 131
management plan 46, 69, 71, 80
management plans 22
medical examination 41
medical model 78
medication 107
memory 52–3, 56, 59, 65
memory changes 17
memory clinic v, 46–7
memory difficulties 38
memory impairment 24
memory loss 41, 47, 59–60, 84,126
memory performance 49
memory test 38, 59
memory testing 28, 52
memory tests v, 34, 41, 63, 87

Index

meningitis 18
mental health officer 156
metabolic causes 14
Mini-Mental State Examination vi, 35, 38, 41, 58, 60, 63, 84
misdiagnosis 2, 33, 50
mobile emergency care schemes 92
MRI brain scans 46, 64
multidisciplinary assessment 4, 47
multidisciplinary patient reviews 92
multi-infarct dementia 9, 49, 53, 55, 97
multiple sclerosis associated dementia 19

N

The NHS and Community Care Act, 1990 136, 157
neoplasia 42, 44
neoplastic 19
nerve growth factor 94, 96
neurofibrillary tangles 10, 12, 1 7
neuroleptic drugs 102
neuroleptic malignant syndrome 103
neuroleptics 79
neurolinguistic programming 111, 113
neurological examination 65
neurotramsitter 95
neurotransmitter deficit 13
NHS and Community Care Act 28
NHS and Community Care Act,1990 1
nihilism 45, 114
nocturnal wandering 105, 128
non-atd dementias v, 17
non-cognitive symptoms 6
non-drug interventions in dementia management vi
non-specific anti-inflammatory drugs 95

non-verbal language 114
nootropics 97
normal pressure hydrocephalus 17, 44
nurse 110, 115
nurse practitioners 87
nurse's role 82–3, 115
nursing home care vi, 78, 88
nutritional causes 14

O

objectivisation 150
occupational therapist 38
occupational therapists 88
oculogyric crisis 103
ongoing bereavement 136, 143
onward referral 45
  to a hospital consultant 46
onward referral of the patients v
orientation 56, 59
orientation aids 117
over-75s assessment profile vi
overdiagnose 34
overdiagnosis 33
overreaction 124

P

a progressive disease v
parathyroid disorders 18
Parkinson's disease 14, 16, 42, 54, 67
parkinsonism 103
pathology v, 9
pathology of ATD 10
patient abuse vi, 148
  family carers 148
  financial abuse 149
  psychological abuse 148
patient's and carers' needs assessment of 69
people with dementia 2, 28
performance anxiety 35
perseveration 23, 40, 120
personalised management plan 4
personality 41
personality change 26, 40

anxiety 27
depression 27
personality changes 26, 142
planned intervention 4
plasma viscosity 64
pneumonia 107
polypharmacy 42
   cause of toxic confusion 42
power of attorney 74, 153
powers of attorney 31
practice nurses 82, 86
presenile dementia 67
primary and secondary tumours 54
primary care team 32, 36, 41, 45, 86, 152
primary cerebral degeneration 14
primary health care team 72, 87
   role in management v, 75
professional 71
prion 19
progressive supranuclear palsy 54
propentofylline 97
pseudodementia 57
psychogeriatric services 48
psychological abuse 148
psychotropic and neuroleptic drug use in dementia vi
psychotropic drugs 102
   extrapyramidal effects 103
psychotropic medication 42

R

reality orientation 83, 88, 114, 116, 118, 124
recreational activities 88, 118
referral to social services 46
refusal of services 151
relative support groups 92
reminiscence 83, 88, 114
reminiscence therapy vi
reminiscence work 114
renal disease 42
residential care 88
residential long-term provision 92
resolution therapies 88
resource management 32
respite care 32, 46, 92, 110, 138, 146, 151-2
role of the nurse 84
roles of the care team vi

S

The Secretaries of State for Health and Social Security 1
selective serotonin re-uptake inhibitors 101
selegeline 96, 106
senile plaques 10, 12-13, 17
serotonin re-uptake inhibitor 130
Sertraline 101
sexual abuse 150
Single photon emission computed tomography 45, 60, 62
sleep 56, 59, 102
sleep disturbance 106
small group therapy 116
social isolation 137, 148
social work department 47, 154-7
Social work department services 90
social work professionals 89
social worker
   role 89
social workers 72, 88
SSRIs 101
standardised assessment 70
standardised assessment criteria 42
stigmatisation 150
stress 134, 143-4
stresses 145, 147
stroke disease 50
subdural haematoma 18
subdural haematomas 44
sundowning 53, 128
support services 67, 142
syndrome 6
syphilis 18, 43
syphilitic serology 43

T

primary and secondary tumours 55
tardive dyskinesia 103
tests of orientation 34
thioridazine 103, 106-7, 127
thyroid 18
thyroid disorder 42
toxic causes 14
toxic damage 20
  alcoholism 20
  aluminium and lead poisoning 20
  solvent abuse 20
toxoplasmosis 18
training for GPs 35
  assessment protocol 35
transient ischaemic attacks 53, 133
trauma 57
trauma and anoxia 14
trazodone 106
treatment of dementia
  nihilistic response 58
tricyclic antidepressants 101
trifluoperazine 103
trust 155
tumours 18
tutor bond 154

U

ultrasonography 64
underdiagnosis 33
urea and electrolytes 43

urinary and faecal incontinence vi
urinary incontinence 139
  management of 131
urinary tract infection 107, 128, 130
urinary tract infections 43, 79
urine dipstick test 43

V

validation 83, 88

validation therapy vi, 114, 116, 118
vascular dementia 9, 15, 16, 64, 108
  caused by 15
  classified into 15
vasodilator drugs 97
visual difficulties 75
vitamin B12 17, 43
vitamin B12 deficiency 54-5
vitamin C 76

W

wandering 53, 123-8, 133, 135, 139, 142, 145
warfarin 108
water and electrolyte disturbance 57
well being 149
Wernicke's encephalopathy 65
Wilson's disease 20
withdrawn behaviour 130

X

x-rays
  chest and skull 62